Hormone Therapy and Replacement in Cancer and Aging-related Diseases

Edited by Leticia B. A. Rangel, Hephzibah Kirubamani, Ian Victor Silva and Paulo Cilas Morais Lyra Junior

Published in London, United Kingdom

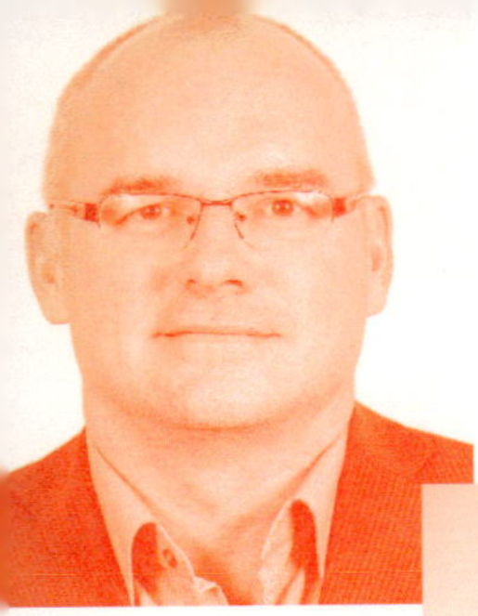
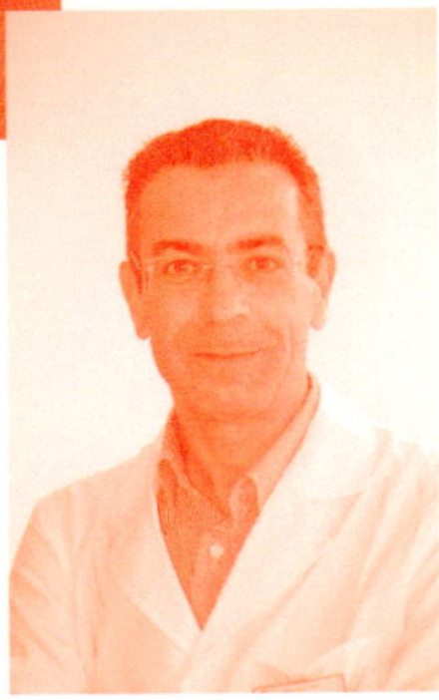
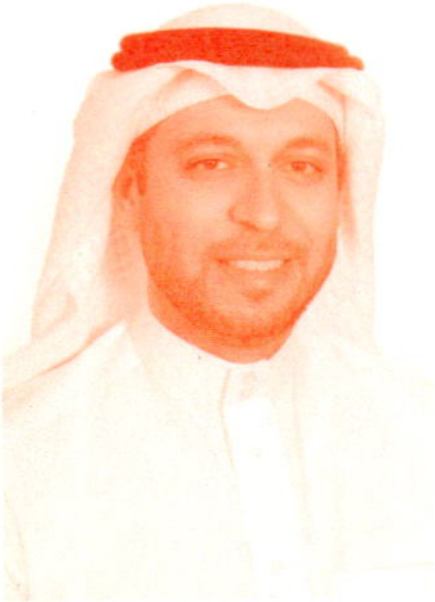
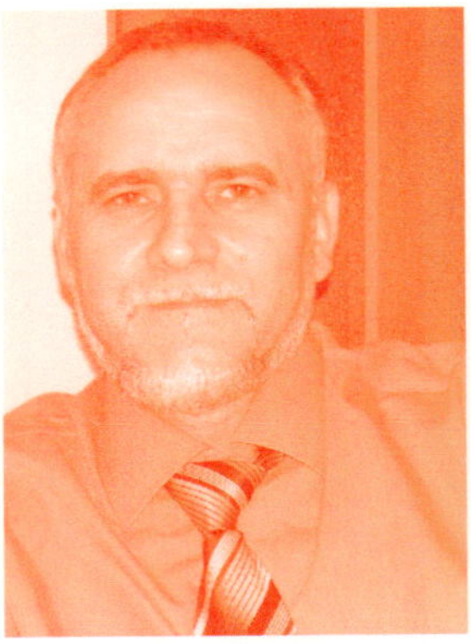
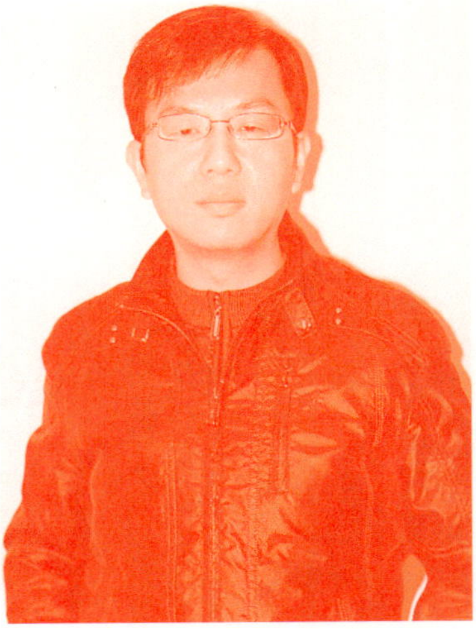
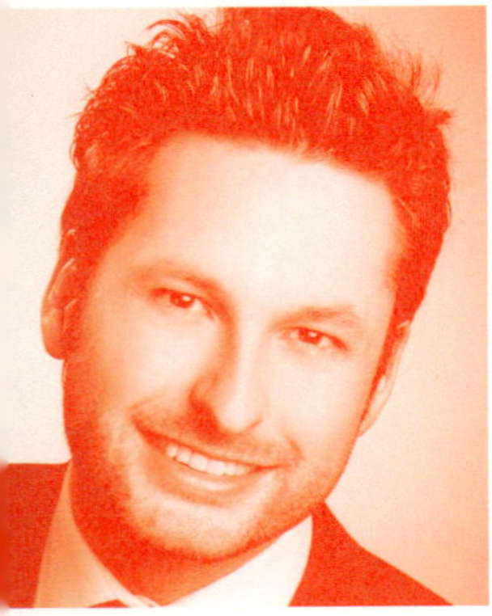
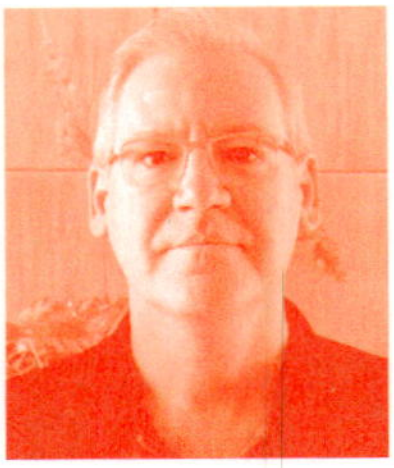

IntechOpen

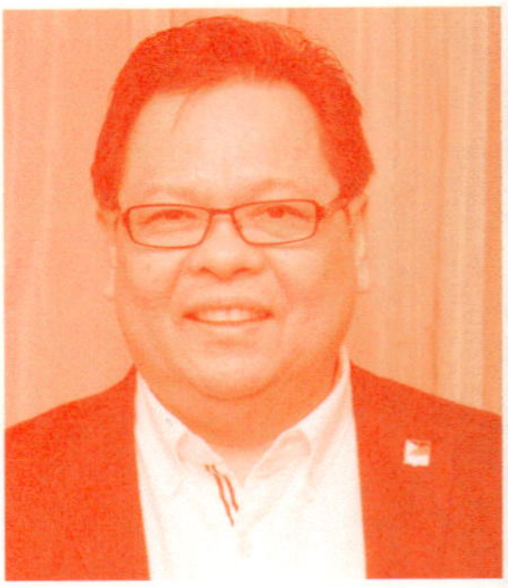
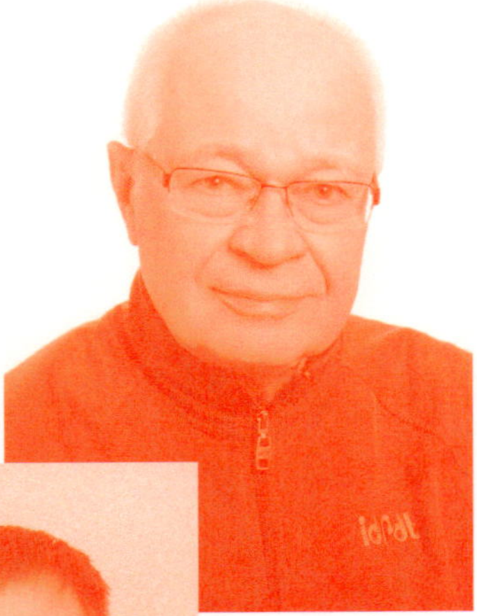
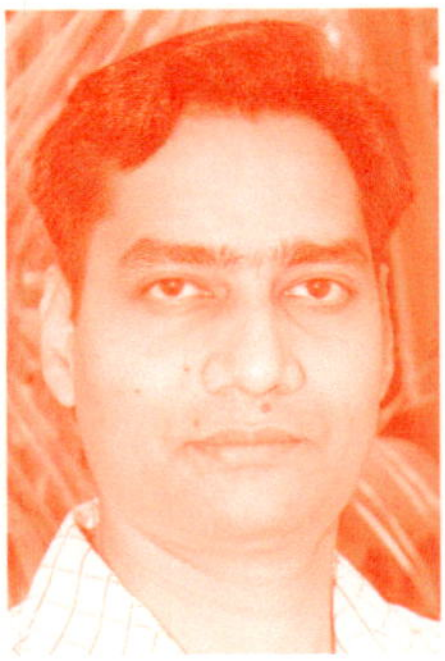
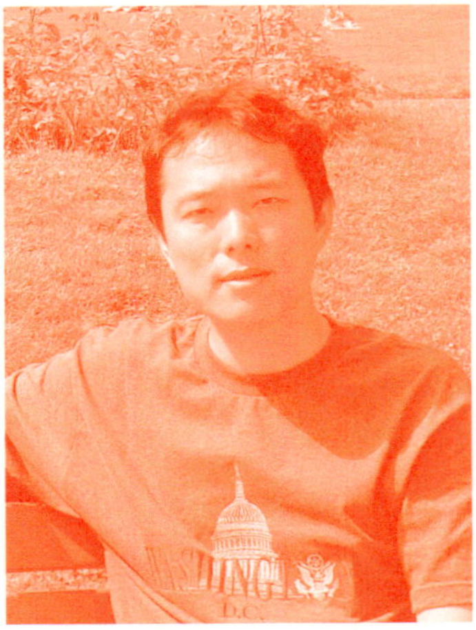
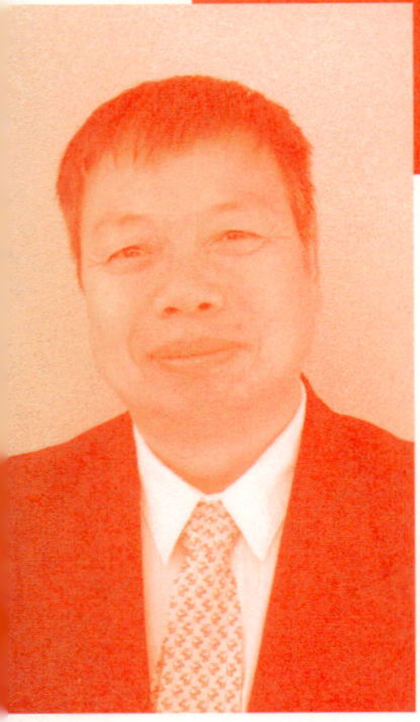
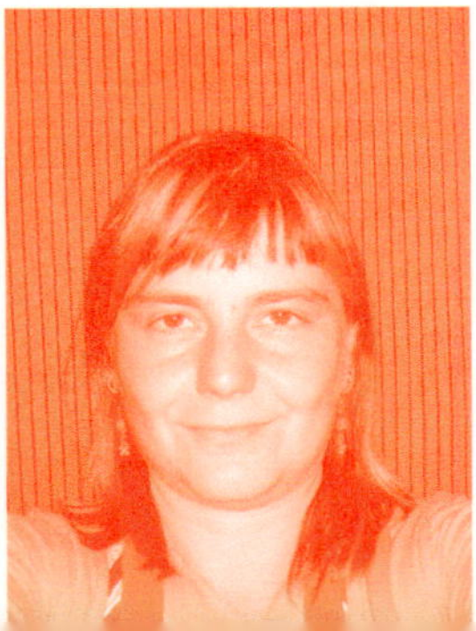

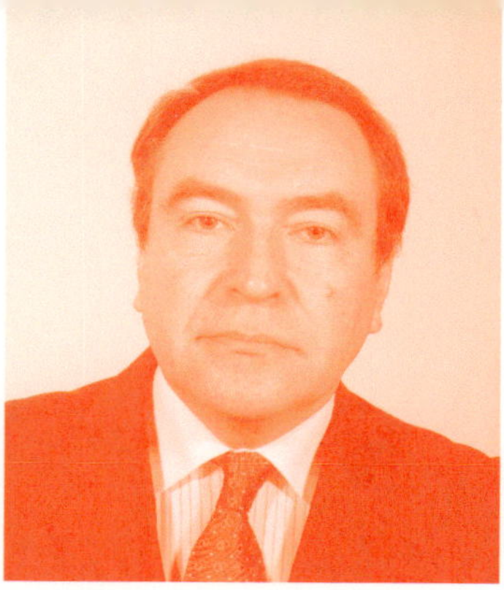
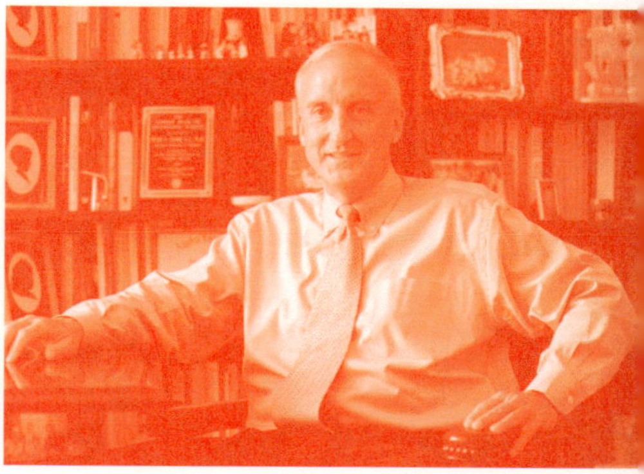
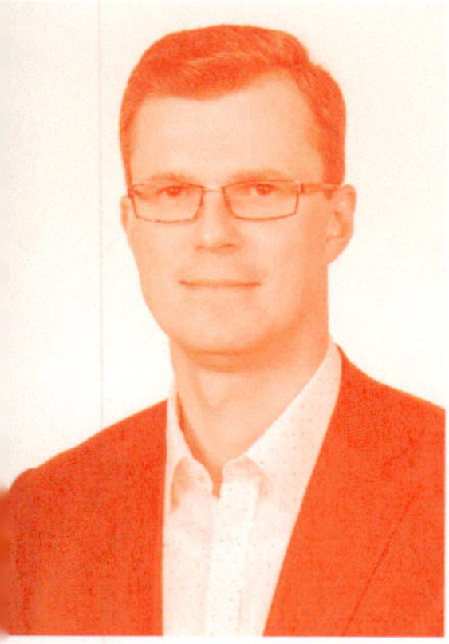
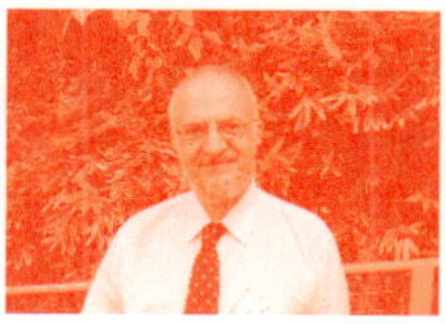
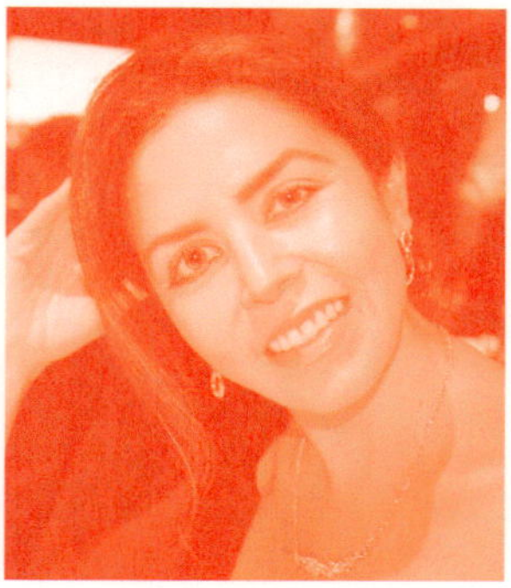

Supporting open minds since 2005

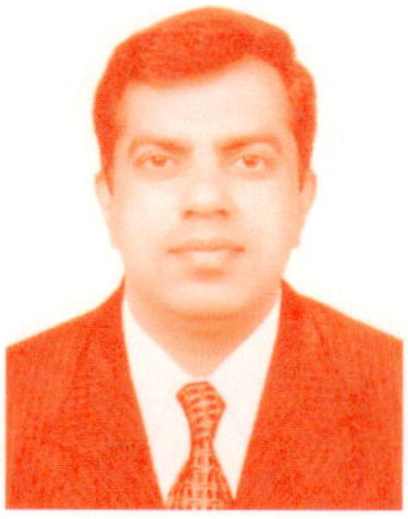
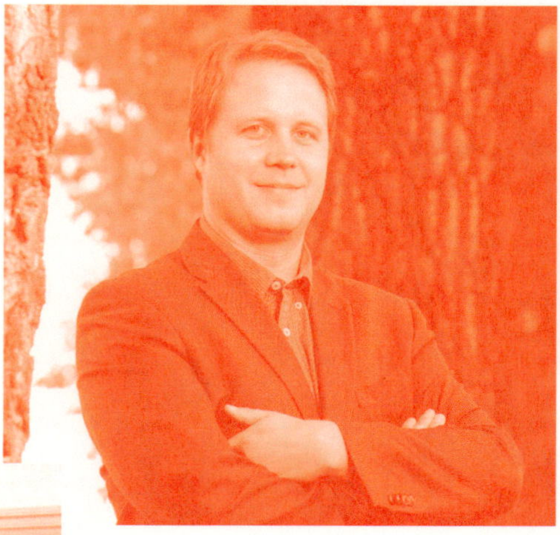
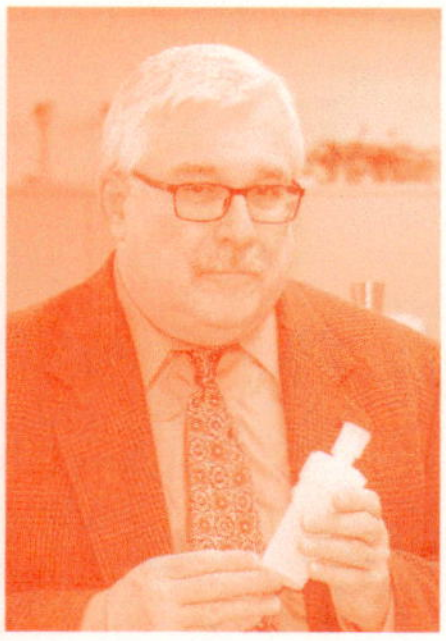
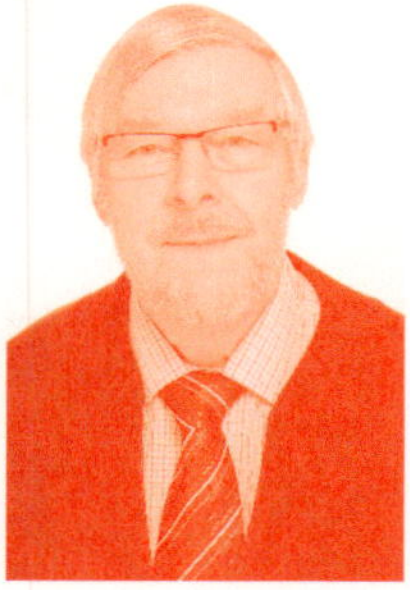
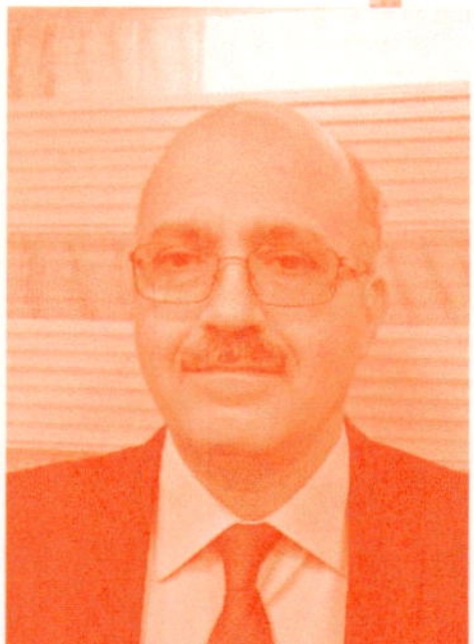
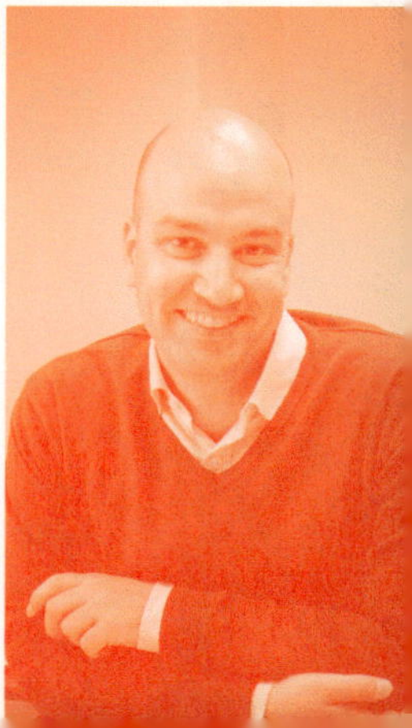
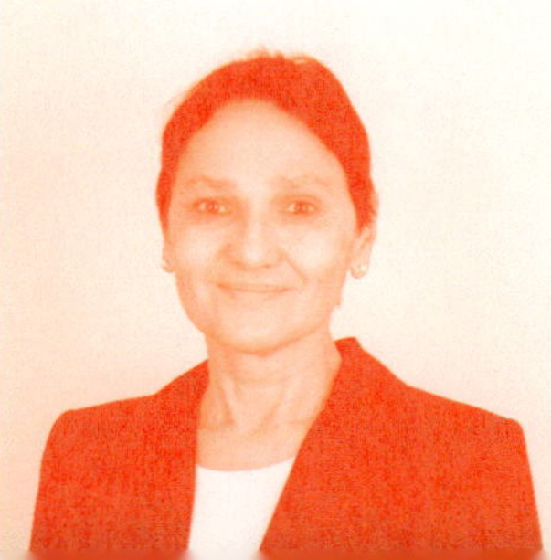

Hormone Therapy and Replacement in Cancer and Aging-related Diseases
http://dx.doi.org/10.5772/intechopen.77810
Edited by Leticia B. A. Rangel, Hephzibah Kirubamani, Ian Victor Silva and Paulo Cilas Morais Lyra Junior

Assistant to the Editor(s): Marcele Mattos De Souza, Diandra Zipinotti Dos Santos

Contributors
Paul Davis, Aleck Hercbergs, Kelly Keating, Hung-Yun Lin, Shaker A Mousa, Geetanjali Tomar, Jay Dave, Sayali Chandekar, Suhas Mhaske, Shaikh Zinnat Ara Nasreen, Elena Usoltseva, Marina Danilova, Manuela Cristina Russu, Hasan Çılgın, Xiaopan Chen, Jing Shu, Jing Zhu, Xiaoyan Guo, Mengxia Ji, Zhizhi Yu, Lili Xing

First published in London, United Kingdom, 2020 by IntechOpen
IntechOpen is the global imprint of INTECHOPEN LIMITED, registered in England and Wales, registration number: 11086078, 7th floor, 10 Lower Thames Street, London, EC3R 6AF, United Kingdom
Printed in Croatia

British Library Cataloguing-in-Publication Data
A catalogue record for this book is available from the British Library

Additional hard and PDF copies can be obtained from orders@intechopen.com

Hormone Therapy and Replacement in Cancer and Aging-related Diseases
Edited by Leticia B. A. Rangel, Hephzibah Kirubamani, Ian Victor Silva and Paulo Cilas Morais Lyra Junior
p. cm.
Print ISBN 978-1-78985-319-3
Online ISBN 978-1-78985-320-9
eBook (PDF) ISBN 978-1-83962-955-6

For EU product safety concerns:
IN TECH d.o.o., Prolaz Marije Krucifikse Kozulić 3, 51000 Rijeka, Croatia, info@intechopen.com or visit our website at intechopen.com.

Meet the editors

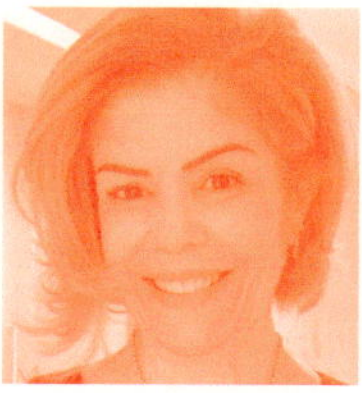

Leticia B. A. Rangel, Pharm.D., Ph.D., is a Full Professor of the Department of Pharmaceutical Sciences, as well as a member of the Biotechnology Program/RENORBIO and the Biochemistry and Pharmacology Program at the Federal University of Espirito Santo (UFES). As the Head of the Laboratory of Cellular and Molecular Biology of Human Cancer, she coordinates projects on ovarian and breast cancers, with emphasis on the cellular and molecular mechanisms of these diseases, the development of biotechnology products and processes, and the discovery of new anticancer molecules. Her scientific network includes the Institute of Biophysics Carlos Chagas Filho (Federal University of Rio de Janeiro), the Division of Clinical Research of the Brazilian National Cancer Institute, The Department of Molecular Medicine, University of Texas at San Antonio (USA), the H. Lee Moffitt Cancer Center (USA), and the Department of Pathology at the John Hopkins University (USA), as well as the private sector. Aside from papers published in international journals, and ongoing patent negotiations, she has been awarded by the Brazilian government in recognition to her contribution in cancer research.

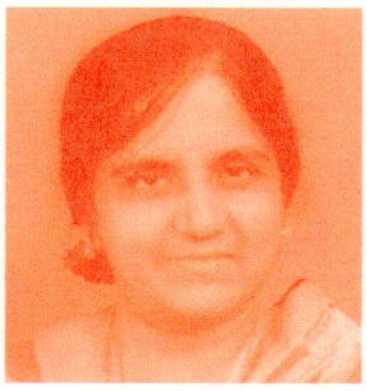

Hephzibah Kirubamani was a former Professor of Obstetrics and Gynecology, Department of Obstetrics and Gynecology, Stanley Medical College, Tamil Nadu Dr. M.G.R. Medical University, since 2006. She was Superintendent of the Government R.S.R.M. Maternity Hospital attached to Stanley Medical College. At present she is a Professor of Obstetrics and Gynecology in the Department of Obstetrics and Gynecology, Saveetha Medical College, SIMATS. She has been teaching undergraduate and postgraduate medical students for 30 years and is an examiner in various universities. She is guiding PhD scholars at Saveetha University, SIMATS. She was instrumental in the Fellowship Programme in Foetal Medicine at Stanley Medical College in 2011. Her field of interest is high-risk pregnancy, emergency obstetrics, and menopause. She has authored the book "Undergraduate Clinical Manual on Obstetrics & Gynaecology" and published many articles in national and international journals. She was a Member of the Academic Council of T.N. Dr.M.G.R. Medical University (2007), Academic Council Member of Saveetha University (2012–2015), and Research Committee Member—India Clen – (2007), Menatshi Medical College (2008), and Indian Menopause Society (2018–2019). She is currently a member and secretary of the Institutional Review Board, Saveetha University. She is past President of the Obstetrics and Gynecology Society of Southern India, and currently Vice President of the Chennai Menopause Society.

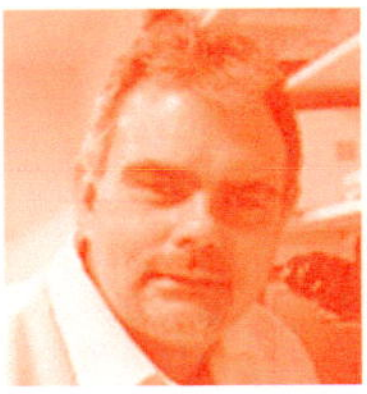

Ian Victor Silva Pharm.D., Ph.D, is a former Associate Professor of the Morphology Department, as well as a member of the Biotechnology/RENORBIO and Biochemistry and Pharmacology Programs of the Health Sciences Center of the Federal University of Espírito Santo where he served as the Head of the Laboratory of Cell Biology of Aging, where he developed studies related to diseases associated with aging in women, such as breast, ovarian, and uterine cancers; Alzheimer's disease; obesity; and osteoporosis. The aim of the referred projects was to develop biotechnological strategies to overcome these diseases, seeking to identify diagnostic, risk, and/or prognostic biomarkers. His scientific network includes Brazilian institutions (INCa, UFRJ, UFSCar, UFRN, UNESP) and foreign institutions (Technion, La Sabana University, The Johns Hopkins University and UTHSCSA). Moreover, he serves as a peer-reviewer in national (RENORBIO, DECIT-SUS, FAPDF, FAPES) and international institutions (Alzheimer's Association).

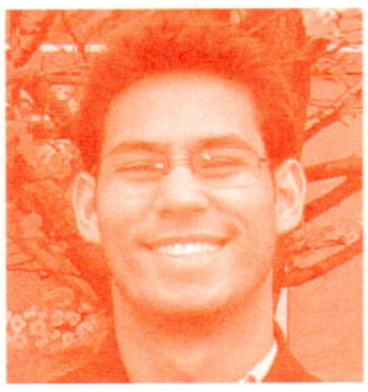

Dr. Paulo Cilas M. Lyra-Jr. is a professor of pharmacology at the Faculty of Education and Environment, Brazil. He obtained his PhD in 2018 from the Federal University of Espírito Santo, Brazil. He worked in collaboration with large consortia, including the NIH-funded Genetic Associations and Mechanisms in Oncology (GAME-ON) consortium, on functional analysis of GWAS hits. He contributed to the functional dissection of the molecular underpinnings of ovarian susceptibility loci, applying molecular techniques, cutting-edge next-generation sequencing, and bioinformatics analysis to map the regulatory landscape at the 8q21 locus. The results were published in *Nature Genetics* (*Nat Genet*. 2019 May;51:815–823). He also contributed to the functional analysis of estrogen-receptor negative breast cancer risk locus (*Nat Genet*. 2017 May;49(5):680– 691).

Contents

Preface XI

Chapter 1 1
Thyroid Hormone Replacement Therapy in Patients with Various Types of Cancer
by Aleck Hercbergs, Paul J. Davis, Hung-Yun Lin, Kelly A. Keating and Shaker A. Mousa

Chapter 2 13
Bone Tumors: Types and Treatments
by Geetanjali B. Tomar, Jay R. Dave, Sayali S. Chandekar and Suhas T. Mhaske

Chapter 3 35
Role of Pineal Hormone Melatonin in a Woman's Life: From Conception to Decline of Life
by Elena N. Usoltseva and Marina V. Danilova

Chapter 4 47
Symptoms of Menopause
by Shaikh Zinnat Ara Nasreen

Chapter 5 55
Endometrial Histology and Safety on Non-Oral Routes of Hormone Therapy for Perimenopausal/Early Menopausal Women: Transdermal Estrogens and Vaginal Micronized Progesterone
by Manuela Cristina Russu

Chapter 6 87
The Role of Hormone Replacement Therapy in the Treatment of Menopausal Symptoms in Patients Diagnosed with Gynecologic Cancer
by Hasan Çilgin

Chapter 7 97
Ovarian Hormonal Change-Related Energy Metabolism and Obesity in Menopausal Women
by Jing Zhu, Mengxia Ji, Lili Xing, Zhizhi Yu, Xiaoyan Guo, Xiaopan Chen and Jing Shu

Preface

This edited volume is a collection of reviewed and relevant research chapters concerning the developments within the hormone therapy and replacement in cancer and aging-related diseases field of study. The book includes scholarly contributions by various authors and is edited by Drs. Leticia Rangel, Hephzibah Kirubamani, Ian Victor Silva, Paulo Cilas Morais Lyra Junior, Marcele Mattos De Souza, and Diandra Zipinotti Dos Santos.

Each contribution comes as a separate chapter complete in itself but directly related to the book's topics and objectives.

The book includes seven chapters, as follows: Thyroid Hormone Replacement Therapy in Patients with Various Types of Cancer; Bone Tumors: Types and Treatments; Role of Pineal Hormone Melatonin in a Woman's Life: From Conception to Decline of Life; Symptoms of Menopause; Endometrial Histology and Safety on Non-Oral Routes of Hormone Therapy for Perimenopausal/Early Menopausal Women: Transdermal Estrogens and Vaginal Micronized Progesterone; The Role of Hormone Replacement Therapy in the Treatment of Menopausal Symptoms in Patients Diagnosed with Gynecologic Cancer; Ovarian Hormonal Change-Related Energy Metabolism and Obesity in Menopausal Women.

The target audience comprises scholars and specialists in the field.

Leticia B. A. Rangel, Pharm. D., PhD.
Full Professor and Investigator,
Head of the Laboratory of Cellular and Molecular Biology of Human Cancer,
Biotechnology Program/RENORBIO,
Biochemistry and Pharmacology Program,
Department of Pharmaceutical Sciences,
Health Sciences Center,
Federal University of Espirito Santo,
Brazil

Chapter 1

Thyroid Hormone Replacement Therapy in Patients with Various Types of Cancer

Aleck Hercbergs, Paul J. Davis, Hung-Yun Lin, Kelly A. Keating and Shaker A. Mousa

Abstract

Primary hypothyroidism is a common endocrine disorder that is effectively treated with L-thyroxine (T4) replacement. Preclinical and limited clinical evidence, however, indicates that T4 is a growth factor for a variety of cancers, acting at the thyroid hormone receptor on plasma membrane integrin αvβ3. T4 is the primary ligand for this receptor, whereas 3,5,3′-triiodo-L-thyronine (T3) is the principal intracellular thyroid hormone analogue. The evidence is reviewed here that T4 is a proliferative for breast, lung, kidney and prostate cancers and for glioblastoma, regulates cancer cell respiration and is a pro-angiogenic factor in established tumors. The recommendation is made that T3 be considered alternative replacement treatment for patients with primary hypothyroidism who also have cancer.

Keywords: thyroid hormone receptors, integrin αvβ3, breast cancer, lung cancer, glioblastoma, renal cell carcinoma

1. Introduction

Spontaneous primary hypothyroidism is a common disorder and prescriptions for L-thyroxine (T4) replacement therapy are among the five most commonly prescribed drugs in the U.S. [1]. The predictable absorbance of T4 from the human gastrointestinal tract and its relatively long half-life in the circulation enable once daily replacement dosing and high patient compliance. 3,5,3′-triiodo-L-thyronine (T3) is also prescribed as thyroid hormone replacement, but its relatively short biologic half-life means that more than once daily dosing is required for replacement.

Integrin αvβ3 is one of a family of plasma membrane proteins that are importantly involved in cell-to-cell and cell-extracellular matrix (ECM) protein interactions that are particularly relevant to tissue structure and function in cancer [2, 3]. αvβ3 is generously expressed by cancer cells and contains a receptor for thyroid hormone at which nongenomic actions of thyroid hormone are initiated [4, 5]. There are no structural homologies between the thyroid hormone receptor site on αvβ3 and the nuclear thyroid hormone receptors (TRs) at which genomic actions of the hormone are initiated [4, 5]. The large panel of genomic actions of T3 that are critical to the function of normal cells in species with thyroid glands involve TRs. T4 is a prohormone for T3 and is not important within cells, except perhaps for regulation of the state of actin [5, 6].

At the cell surface receptor for thyroid hormone on αvβ3, T4 is the principal ligand [7, 8] and has at physiological concentrations a set of actions that include cancer cell proliferation [4, 5], cancer cell defense pathways, e.g., anti-apoptosis [5], and the fostering of tumor-relevant angiogenesis [9, 10]. In nonmalignant cells, the T4 receptor on αvβ3 may have certain specific functions in neurons during development [11, 12], in phagocytosis [13] and in platelet aggregation [14]. Studies *in vitro* have disclosed that T4 stimulates the proliferation of breast cancer cells [15–17], lung cancer [18, 19] and kidney cancer [20] cells, glioblastoma cells [8, 21] and other tumor cells [22]. Pharmacologic blockade of T4 action at the integrin is feasible with tetraiodothyroacetic acid (tetrac) and modified forms of tetrac [7, 17, 20, 23–26] arrest tumor xenografts.

In patients with a variety of advanced solid tumors, elimination of endogenous T4 and substitution of exogenous T3 ("euthyroid hypothyroxinemia") has also been shown to arrest tumor growth [27]. Other earlier studies of pharmacologic induction of mild hypothyroidism (decreased circulating host T4 without T3 replacement) may also improve survival in patients with glioblastoma [27] and renal cell carcinoma [28]. The aggressive behavior of certain cancers may also be ameliorated in the setting of spontaneous hypothyroidism [29].

In this chapter, we will extend our discussion of the possibility that clinical behaviors of a number of cancers are supported by endogenous T4 or exogenous T4 replacement in cancer patients who have concurrent hypothyroidism [16, 27, 29, 30]. In addition to the general principle that proliferation of many types of cancer cells is reduced by concurrent hypothyroidism, there are examples of highly specific roles that T4 may play in the behavior of certain tumors. In estrogen receptor-positive (ER^+) cancer cells, T4 stimulates mitogen-activated protein kinase (MAPK)-dependent, specific phosphorylation of ERα in the absence of estrogen [15]. This may also apply to lung cancer cells that express ER. In the postmenopausal patient with such ER-expressing tumors, host T4 may substitute for host estrogen.

We also will review actions of T4 that appear to be relevant to chemoresistance and to radioresistance. The chemoresistance role played by T4 may involve (a) specific antagonism of chemotherapeutic drug-induced apoptosis in tumor cells or (b) enhanced export by tumor cells of cancer treatment agents [31]. Integrin αvβ3 is substantially involved in the induction of radioresistance in tumor cells [32–34], and the thyroid hormone receptor on αvβ3 controls the contribution of the integrin to radioresistance.

We conclude that for T4-treated patients with primary hypothyroidism who develop aggressive cancers, it is worthwhile to consider elimination of replacement T4 and management of hypothyroidism with T3.

2. Breast cancer

The published MD Anderson Cancer Center experience with breast cancer patients who develop spontaneous hypothyroidism is that the latter state changes the course of the cancer, i.e., the disease is less aggressive [29]. The survival of patients with end-stage metastatic breast cancer may be lengthened by induction of the state of euthyroid hypothyroxinemia [27]. Chemically modified tetrac that acts at the thyroid hormone receptor on αvβ3 significantly reduces breast cancer xenograft size in the nude mouse [24].

An extensive survey of survival pathway gene transcription in triple-negative human (MDA-MB-231) breast cancer cells revealed that the thyroid hormone receptor on αvβ3 differentially regulated expression of genes for anti-apoptotic X-linked inhibitor of apoptosis (XIAP), myeloid cell leukemia-1 (MCL-1), and for pro-apoptotic caspase-2 (CASP2) and BCL2L14 [26]. Acting in an anticancer mode, tetrac in this study downregulated anti-apoptotic genes and increased expression of pro-apoptotic genes. The thyroid hormone receptor on integrin αvβ3 also affected breast cancer genes linked to angiogenesis. In addition, T4 and chemically modified tetrac (nano-diamino-tetrac, NDAT) stimulate and inhibit, respectively, programmed death ligand-1 (PD-L1) gene expression in cultured MDA-MB-231 breast cancer cells [17].

The observation 10 years ago that tetrac enhanced tumor cell uptake of doxorubicin, cisplatin and other chemotherapeutic agents suggested that a cell export system was regulated from integrin αvβ3 in breast cancer cells [35]. It was subsequently shown that activity of the p-glycoprotein (P-gp) plasma membrane efflux pump was regulated by thyroid hormone analogues that are acting at αvβ3 [31]. The implication of the observations is that T4 may act at the integrin to enhance P-gp action. Such an action may be desirable in healthy, nonmalignant cells for ridding the cells of toxic substances; in cancer cells, the action supports chemoresistance.

Radioresistance of certain cancer cells can be induced rapidly by X-radiation via a change in conformation of integrin αvβ3 [32, 33], but this has not yet been examined in breast cancer cells. The STAT3 [36] and NF-κB [37] signal transduction pathways appear to be involved in the development of radioresistance in breast cancer cells, and both of these signaling molecules are regulated via integrin αvβ3 and the thyroid hormone receptor [5, 38].

Taken individually and together, the breast cancer-focused actions of T4 that are initiated at the iodothyronine receptor on integrin αvβ3 are reason to consider in patients with breast cancer and primary hypothyroidism a modification of standard replacement therapy with T4. The alternative approaches are T3 replacement or reduction in T4 dosage that permits endogenous thyroid-stimulating hormone (TSH) elevation without symptoms of hypothyroidism.

3. Prostate cancer

An anti-thryoid agent, propylthiouracil (PTU), inhibited the growth of xenografts in nude mice of two human prostate cancer cell lines [39]. No direct effect of PTU on the tumor cells was found *in vitro*. PTU reduces circulating levels of both T4 and T3. In a study conducted in smokers, overt spontaneous hypothyroidism was associated with a decreased risk of prostate cancer, as was elevation of circulating TSH [40]. Increased TSH presumptively reflected patient-specific decreases within the normal range of circulating T4 and T3 (latent hypothyroidism). The authors speculated that the reduced risk of prostate cancer risk was related to decreased T4 action at integrin αvβ3. In another study, latent hypothyroidism was a predictive marker of positive response in patients with prostate cancer undergoing a specific therapy (abiraterone acetate) [41].

Preclinical studies of iodothyronines in prostate cancer xenografts and of possible contributions of integrin αvβ3 to prostate cancer have not yet been reported. However, αvβ3 response to X-radiation has been examined in prostate cancer (PC3) cells *in vitro* [32]. Activation of the integrin was induced by radiation and this response was prevented by tetrac, implicating the thyroid hormone receptor on the integrin in the defensive response.

4. Lung cancer

Human non-small cell (NCI-H522) lung carcinoma cells and small cell (NCI-H510A) cancer cells proliferate *in vitro* in response to physiological concentrations of T4 and supraphysiological levels of T3 [19]. Tetrac inhibited these responses, implicating the thyroid hormone receptor on integrin αvβ3 in the response. These cell lines express ERα As is the case in human breast cancer cells that express ER, the estrogen receptor is subject to activation/phosphorylation in the presence of T4. ER activation is associated with cancer cell proliferation quantitated by PCNA expression and thymidine incorporation. The specific ERα antagonist compound, ICI 182,770, diminished the activation by T4 of the estrogen receptor, as well as the stimulation of proliferation by T4. The growth of non-small cell (H1299) lung carcinoma xenografts is reversed by unmodified and chemically modified tetrac [23], consistent with a critical role for αvβ3 in the regulation of tumor growth.

More information available about T4 action on lung cancer is limited. Euthyroid hypothyroxinemia appears to slow the course of metastatic lung carcinoma [27].

5. Glioblastoma

In preclinical studies, T4 has been shown to be a growth factor for gliomas [21], and the actions of chemically modified tetrac molecules at the thyroid hormone receptor on integrin αvβ3 significantly increased transcription of a panel of pro-apoptotic genes (*p53*, *p21*, *PIG*, *BAD*) [7]. The latter results imply that T4 action at the integrin may undesirably either decease or not affect expression of these genes. In a limited *in vitro* study, T3 restricted glioblastoma cell proliferation [42] and preclinical studies have also shown that NDAT—which limits access of T4 to its receptor on integrin αvβ3 on tumor cells—suppresses growth and is anti-angiogenic in glioblastoma xenografts [25].

In 2003, chemical induction of mild hypothyroidism with propylthiouracil (PTU) was shown in patients with recurrent, high-grade glioblastoma to be associated with significant prolongation of survival [43]. More recently, euthyroid hypothyroxinemia has significantly extended survival in patients with end-stage glioblastoma [27].

Induction of euthyroid hypothyroxinemia has been effective in prolonging survival of the few glioblastoma patients with end-stage disease in whom it has been tested [27].

6. Renal cell carcinoma

Among the side effects of chemotherapeutic tyrosine kinase inhibitors (TKIs) used in management of renal cell carcinoma (RCC) is induction of preclinical primary hypothyroidism. The "preclinical" state is an elevation of circulating TSH with normal range serum T4 and T3 concentrations. An extensive clinical literature documents that response of metastatic RCC to TKIs sorafenib and sunitinib is importantly enhanced when drug-induced hypothyroidism complicates tumor management [28, 30, 44–48]. TKIs may cause hypothyroidism in up to 40% of treated patients. The therapeutic response to the recognition of drug-induced preclinical primary hypothyroidism in RCC patients was administration of exogenous T4 to the point of returning host TSH to the normal range. In the noncancerous patient with preclinical hypothyroidism, the American Thyroid Association has endorsed a strategy of replacement thyroid hormone as needed to prevent symptoms of hypothyroidism and maintain serum TSH below 10 mIU/mL [49]. This approach may be adequate to take advantage of the TKI support that preclinical hypothyroidism provides with reduction in circulating T4 within the normal range.

The relevance of the thyroid hormone receptor on integrin αvβ3 to RCC has been shown in xenograft studies in the nude mouse [20]. Tetrac and chemically modified tetrac significantly reduced xenograft volume and xenograft vascularity in 20-day studies.

The clinical and preclinical information available on RCC documents the importance of thyroid hormone to RCC. When drug-induced or spontaneous early hypothyroidism complicates the course of RCC, substantial decision-making surrounds when and with what hormone the hypothyroid state should be addressed.

7. Pancreatic carcinoma

Pancreatic cancer is an aggressive tumor locally and metastasizes regionally and systemically with sufficient frequency to have a very unsatisfactory 5-year survival. The relevance of thyroid hormone to tumor behavior has been shown in xenograft studies [50]. Unmodified and chemically modified tetrac in 15-day studies reduced xenograft size by up to 50% and reduced graft vascularity. Tumor gene expression studies showed that chemically modified tetrac acted via αvβ3 to reduce epidermal growth factor receptor (EGFR) gene and anti-apoptotic XIAP gene transcription and to increase expression of pro-apoptotic p53 and anti-angiogenic thrombospondin 1. The implication of these results is that T4—whose binding to αvβ3 is inhibited by tetrac—may play an important tumor support role in this form of cancer.

In contrast to RCC, there is not a significant literature on chemotherapeutic drug-induced hypothyroidism in patients with pancreatic carcinoma. Induction of euthyroid hypothyroxinemia appears to slow the course of advanced pancreatic cancer [27].

8. Discussion

At the cancer cell surface receptor for thyroid hormone on the extracellular domain of integrin αvβ3, T4 is an active hormone, supporting a variety of critical tumor cell functions [5, 10, 26]. In contrast, T4 within normal cells and cancer cells can serve as a prohormone source for T3. T4 is the standard of care for management of hypothyroidism [49].

A small minority of hypothyroid patients coincidentally have an experience with cancer of various types, as pointed out above. The behavior of the tumors is reported in most clinical studies of this combination of diseases to be less aggressive. But interpretation of the data is sometimes difficult because a distinction may not be made between T4-treated and untreated spontaneous hypothyroid states and the appearance or behavior of the cancer. However, substantial information is now available about the link of hypothyroid state to tumor behavior in those patients in whom hypothyroidism is a side effect of chemotherapy, e.g., TKI use in RCC patients [28, 47, 51], or the clinical use of euthyroid hypothyroxinemia in patients with advanced cancers [27].

A body of preclinical evidence also exists to indicate that T4 stimulates proliferation of a variety of tumors, and this effect is initiated at a plasma membrane receptor for thyroid hormone that is generously expressed in cancer cells [5]. At this receptor site, T4 is also anti-apoptotic [5] and supports tumor-relevant angiogenesis [5]. The integrin may also be involved in tumor cell radioresistance [32, 33].

Against this background, we raise the issue of whether prescription of T4 replacement in hypothyroid patients with concurrent cancer should be routine. T3 is not active at physiological concentrations at the integrin receptor for thyroid hormone and we have shown that T3 can be substituted for endogenous T4 in euthyroid patients with cancer with a result of improved survival and, in some cases, reduction in tumor size. Thus, we feel that the use of T3 replacement can be endorsed in patients with spontaneous or TKI-induced hypothyroidism and cancer. A disadvantage is that T3 must be administered more than once daily because of its short half-life.

A particularly interesting example of the complexity of the relationships of thyroid hormone and cancer is the capacity of T4 to activate ERα in ER-positive breast cancer cells in the absence of estrogen [15]. In addition, T4 is able to promote trafficking of ER from cytoplasm to nucleus [52]. Thus, ER in breast cancer of the postmenopausal euthyroid woman remains a functional component of the tumor.

The setting of thyroid cancer and concomitant hypothyroidism management is not included in the sections above in this review but has been discussed elsewhere by the current authors [53]. Hypothyroidism in the setting of thyroid cancer may of course be a consequence of radiation therapy of the tumor. Exogenous T4 may be administered in patients with thyroid cancers to suppress endogenous thyrotropin (TSH) that may support thyroid tumor cell proliferation. What we have recommended in the context of thyroid cancer and hypothyroidism or T4-suppression of endogenous TSH with T4 and intractable tumor behavior is that the use of T3 be considered [53] as, respectively, hormone replacement or vehicle to suppress host TSH.

Author details

Aleck Hercbergs[1], Paul J. Davis[2,3]*, Hung-Yun Lin[4,5,6,7], Kelly A. Keating[3] and Shaker A. Mousa[3]

1 Department of Radiation Oncology, The Cleveland Clinic, Cleveland, OH, USA

2 Department of Medicine, Albany Medical College, Albany, NY, USA

3 Pharmaceutical Research Institute, Albany College of Pharmacy and Health Sciences, Rensselaer, NY, USA

4 Taipei Cancer Center, Taipei, Taiwan

5 Graduate Institute for Cancer Molecular Biology and Drug Discovery, Taipei, Taiwan

6 Traditional Herbal Medicine Research Center of Taipei Medical University Hospital, Taipei, Taiwan

7 TMU Research Center of Cancer Translational Medicine, Taipei Medical University, Taipei, Taiwan

*Address all correspondence to: pdavis.ordwayst@gmail.com

References

[1] Fuentes AV, Pineda MD, Venkata KCN. Comprehension of top 200 prescribed drugs in the US as a resource for pharmacy teaching, training and practice. Pharmacy (Basel). 2018;**6**:43. DOI: 10.3390/pharmacy6020043

[2] Seguin L, Desgrosellier JS, Weis SM, Cheresh DA. Integrins and cancer: Regulators of cancer stemness, metastasis, and drug resistance. Trends in Cell Biology. 2015;**25**:234-240. DOI: 10.1016/j.tcb.2014.12.006

[3] Desgrosellier JS, Cheresh DA. Integrins in cancer: Biological implications and therapeutic opportunities. Nature Reviews Cancer. 2010;**10**:9-22. DOI: 10.1038/nrc2748

[4] Cheng SY, Leonard JL, Davis PJ. Molecular aspects of thyroid hormone actions. Endocrine Reviews. 2010;**31**:139-170. DOI: 10.1210/er.2009-0007

[5] Lin HY, Chin YT, Yang YC, Lai HY, Wang-Peng J, Liu LF, et al. Thyroid hormone, cancer, and apoptosis. Comprehensive Physiology. 2016;**6**:1221-1237. DOI: 10.1002/cphy.c150035

[6] Farwell AP, Leonard JL. Extranuclear actions of thyroid hormone in the brain. In: Porterfield SP, Hendrich CE, editors. Recent Research Developments in Neuroendocrinology—Thyroid Hormone and Brain Maturation. Trivandrum, India: Research Signpost; 1997. pp. 113-130

[7] Lin HY, Landersdorfer CB, London D, Meng R, Lim CU, Lin C, et al. Pharmacodynamic modeling of anti-cancer activity of tetraiodothyroacetic acid in a perfused cell culture system. PLoS Computational Biology. 2011;7:e1001073. DOI: 10.1371/journal.pcbi.1001073

[8] Lin HY, Sun M, Tang HY, Lin C, Luidens MK, Mousa SA, et al. L-Thyroxine vs. 3,5,3′-triiodo-L-thyronine and cell proliferation: Activation of mitogen-activated protein kinase and phosphatidylinositol 3-kinase. American Journal of Physiology. Cell Physiology. 2009;**296**:C980-C991. DOI: 10.1152/ajpcell.00305.2008

[9] Davis PJ, Sudha T, Lin HY, Mousa SA. Thyroid hormone, hormone analogs, and angiogenesis. Comprehensive Physiology. 2015;**6**:353-362. DOI: 10.1002/cphy.c150011

[10] Mousa SA, Lin HY, Tang HY, Hercbergs A, Luidens MK, Davis PJ. Modulation of angiogenesis by thyroid hormone and hormone analogues: Implications for cancer management. Angiogenesis. 2014;**17**:463-469. DOI: 10.1007/s10456-014-9418-5

[11] Yonkers MA, Ribera AB. Sensory neuron sodium current requires nongenomic actions of thyroid hormone during development. Journal of Neurophysiology. 2008;**100**:2719-2725. DOI: 10.1152/jn.90801.2008

[12] Yonkers MA, Ribera AB. Molecular components underlying nongenomic thyroid hormone signaling in embryonic zebrafish neurons. Neural Development. 2009;**4**:20. DOI: 10.1186/1749-8104-4-20

[13] Chen Y, Sjolinder M, Wang X, Altenbacher G, Hagner M, Berglund P, et al. Thyroid hormone enhances nitric oxide-mediated bacterial clearance and promotes survival after meningococcal infection. PLoS ONE. 2012;**7**:e41445. DOI: 10.1371/journal.pone.0041445

[14] Mousa SS, Davis FB, Davis PJ, Mousa SA. Human platelet aggregation and degranulation is

induced in vitro by L-thyroxine, but not by 3,5,3′-triiodo-L-thyronine or diiodothyropropionic acid (DITPA). Clinical and Applied Thrombosis/Hemostasis. 2010;**16**:288-293. DOI: 10.1177/1076029609348315

[15] Tang HY, Lin HY, Zhang S, Davis FB, Davis PJ. Thyroid hormone causes mitogen-activated protein kinase-dependent phosphorylation of the nuclear estrogen receptor. Endocrinology. 2004;**145**:3265-3272. DOI: 10.1210/en.2004-0308

[16] Hercbergs A, Mousa SA, Leinung M, Lin HY, Davis PJ. Thyroid hormone in the clinic and breast cancer. Hormones & Cancer. 2018;**9**:139-143. DOI: 10.1007/s12672-018-0326-9

[17] Lin HY, Chin YT, Nana AW, Shih YJ, Lai HY, Tang HY, et al. Actions of L-thyroxine and Nano-diamino-tetrac (Nanotetrac) on PD-L1 in cancer cells. Steroids. 2016;**114**:59-67. DOI: 10.1016/j.steroids.2016.05.006

[18] Davis PJ, Davis FB, Mousa SA, Luidens MK, Lin HY. Membrane receptor for thyroid hormone: Physiologic and pharmacologic implications. Annual Review of Pharmacology and Toxicology. 2011;**51**:99-115. DOI: 10.1146/annurev-pharmtox-010510-100512

[19] Meng R, Tang HY, Westfall J, London D, Cao JH, Mousa SA, et al. Crosstalk between integrin αvβ3 and estrogen receptor-α is involved in thyroid hormone-induced proliferation in human lung carcinoma cells. PLoS ONE. 2011;**6**:e27547. DOI: 10.1371/journal.pone.0027547

[20] Yalcin M, Bharali DJ, Lansing L, Dyskin E, Mousa SS, Hercbergs A, et al. Tetraidothyroacetic acid (tetrac) and tetrac nanoparticles inhibit growth of human renal cell carcinoma xenografts. Anticancer Research. 2009;**29**:3825-3831

[21] Davis FB, Tang HY, Shih A, Keating T, Lansing L, Hercbergs A, et al. Acting via a cell surface receptor, thyroid hormone is a growth factor for glioma cells. Cancer Research. 2006;**66**:7270-7275. DOI: 10.1158/0008-5472.CAN-05-4365

[22] Fabian ID, Rosner M, Fabian I, Vishnevskia-Dai V, Zloto O, Shinderman Maman E, et al. Low thyroid hormone levels improve survival in murine model for ocular melanoma. Oncotarget. 2015;**6**:11038-11046. DOI: 10.18632/oncotarget.3566

[23] Mousa SA, Yalcin M, Bharali DJ, Meng R, Tang HY, Lin HY, et al. Tetraiodothyroacetic acid and its nanoformulation inhibit thyroid hormone stimulation of non-small cell lung cancer cells in vitro and its growth in xenografts. Lung Cancer. 2012;**76**:39-45. DOI: 10.1016/j.lungcan.2011.10.003

[24] Bharali DJ, Yalcin M, Davis PJ, Mousa SA. Tetraiodothyroacetic acid-conjugated PLGA nanoparticles: A nanomedicine approach to treat drug-resistant breast cancer. Nanomedicine (London, England). 2013;**8**:1943-1954. DOI: 10.2217/nnm.12.200

[25] Sudha T, Bharali DJ, Sell S, Darwish NHE, Davis PJ, Mousa SA. Nanoparticulate tetrac inhibits growth and vascularity of glioblastoma xenografts. Hormones & Cancer. 2017;**8**:157-165. DOI: 10.1007/s12672-017-0293-6

[26] Glinskii AB, Glinsky GV, Lin HY, Tang HY, Sun M, Davis FB, et al. Modification of survival pathway gene expression in human breast cancer cells by tetraiodothyroacetic acid (tetrac). Cell Cycle. 2009;**8**:3562-3570. DOI: 10.4161/cc.8.21.9963

[27] Hercbergs A, Johnson RE, Ashur-Fabian O, Garfield DH, Davis PJ.

Medically induced euthyroid hypothyroxinemia may extend survival in compassionate need cancer patients: An observational study. The Oncologist. 2015;**20**:72-76. DOI: 10.1634/theoncologist.2014-0308

[28] Schmidinger M, Vogl UM, Bojic M, Lamm W, Heinzl H, Haitel A, et al. Hypothyroidism in patients with renal cell carcinoma: Blessing or curse? Cancer. 2011;**117**:534-544. DOI: 10.1002/cncr.25422

[29] Cristofanilli M, Yamamura Y, Kau SW, Bevers T, Strom S, Patangan M, et al. Thyroid hormone and breast carcinoma. Primary hypothyroidism is associated with a reduced incidence of primary breast carcinoma. Cancer. 2005;**103**:1122-1128. DOI: 10.1002/cncr.20881

[30] Riesenbeck LM, Bierer S, Hoffmeister I, Kopke T, Papavassilis P, Hertle L, et al. Hypothyroidism correlates with a better prognosis in metastatic renal cancer patients treated with sorafenib or sunitinib. World Journal of Urology. 2011;**29**:807-813. DOI: 10.1007/s00345-010-0627-2

[31] Davis PJ, Incerpi S, Lin HY, Tang HY, Sudha T, Mousa SA. Thyroid hormone and P-glycoprotein in tumor cells. BioMed Research International. 2015;**2015**:168427. DOI: 10.1155/2015/168427

[32] Leith JT, Hercbergs A, Kenney S, Mousa SA, Davis PJ. Activation of tumor cell integrin αvβ3 by radiation and reversal of activation by chemically modified tetraiodothyroacetic acid (tetrac). Endocrine Research. 2018;**43**:215-219. DOI: 10.1080/07435800.2018.1456550

[33] Leith JT, Mousa SA, Hercbergs A, Lin HY, Davis PJ. Radioresistance of cancer cells, integrin αvβ3 and thyroid hormone. Oncotarget. 2018;**9**:37069-37075. DOI: 10.18632/oncotarget.26434

[34] Leith JT, Davis PJ, Mousa SA, Hercbergs AA. In vitro effects of tetraiodothyroacetic acid combined with X-irradiation on basal cell carcinoma cells. Cell Cycle. 2017;**16**:367-373. DOI: 10.1080/15384101.2016.1269044

[35] Rebbaa A, Chu F, Davis FB, Davis PJ, Mousa SA. Novel function of the thyroid hormone analog tetraiodothyroacetic acid: A cancer chemosensitizing and anti-cancer agent. Angiogenesis. 2008;**11**:269-276. DOI: 10.1007/s10456-008-9110-8

[36] Kim JS, Kim HA, Seong MK, Seol H, Oh JS, Kim EK, et al. STAT3-survivin signaling mediates a poor response to radiotherapy in HER2-positive breast cancers. Oncotarget. 2016;**7**:7055-7065. DOI: 10.18632/oncotarget.6855

[37] Veuger SJ, Hunter JE, Durkacz BW. Ionizing radiation-induced NF-κB activation requires PARP-1 function to confer radioresistance. Oncogene. 2009;**28**:832-842. DOI: 10.1038/onc.2008.439

[38] Zhao Y, Tan Y, Meng T, Liu X, Zhu Y, Hong Y, et al. Simultaneous targeting therapy for lung metastasis and breast tumor by blocking the NF-κB signaling pathway using celastrol-loaded micelles. Drug Delivery. 2018;**25**:341-352. DOI: 10.1080/10717544.2018.1425778

[39] Theodossiou C, Schwarzenberger P. Propylthiouracil reduces xenograft tumor growth in an athymic nude mouse prostate cancer model. The American Journal of the Medical Sciences. 2000;**319**:96-99

[40] Mondul AM, Weinstein SJ, Bosworth T, Remaley AT, Virtamo J, Albanes D. Circulating thyroxine, thyroid-stimulating hormone, and hypothyroid status and the risk of prostate cancer. PLoS ONE.

2012;**7**:e47730. DOI: 10.1371/journal.pone.0047730

[41] Heidegger I, Nagele U, Pircher A, Pichler R, Horninger W, Bektic J. Latent hypothyreosis as a clinical biomarker for therapy response under abiraterone acetate therapy. Anticancer Research. 2014;**34**:307-311

[42] Liappas A, Mourouzis I, Zisakis A, Economou K, Lea RW, Pantos C. Cell-type-dependent thyroid hormone effects on glioma tumor cell lines. Journal of Thyroid Research. 2011;**2011**:856050. DOI: 10.4061/2011/856050

[43] Hercbergs AA, Goyal LK, Suh JH, Lee S, Reddy CA, Cohen BH, et al. Propylthiouracil-induced chemical hypothyroidism with high-dose tamoxifen prolongs survival in recurrent high grade glioma: A phase I/II study. Anticancer Research. 2003;**23**:617-626

[44] Buda-Nowak A, Kucharz J, Dumnicka P, Kuzniewski M, Herman RM, Zygulska AL, et al. Sunitinib-induced hypothyroidism predicts progression-free survival in metastatic renal cell carcinoma patients. Medical Oncology. 2017;**34**:68. DOI: 10.1007/s12032-017-0928-z

[45] Song Y, Du C, Zhang W, Sun Y, Yang L, Cui C, et al. A study on the association between hyperlipidemia and hypothyroidism and the response to TKIs in metastatic renal cell carcinoma. Asia-Pacific Journal of Clinical Oncology. 2016;**12**:174-180. DOI: 10.1111/ajco.12473

[46] Bozkurt O, Karaca H, Hacibekiroglu I, Kaplan MA, Duzkopru Y, Uysal M, et al. Is sunitinib-induced hypothyroidism a predictive clinical marker for better response in metastatic renal cell carcinoma patients? Journal of Chemotherapy. 2016;**28**:230-234. DOI: 10.1179/1973947815Y.0000000039

[47] Bailey EB, Tantravahi SK, Poole A, Agarwal AM, Straubhar AM, Batten JA, et al. Correlation of degree of hypothyroidism with survival outcomes in patients with metastatic renal cell carcinoma receiving vascular endothelial growth factor receptor tyrosine kinase inhibitors. Clinical Genitourinary Cancer. 2015;**13**:e131-e137. DOI: 10.1016/j.clgc.2014.11.002

[48] Kappers MH, van Esch JH, Smedts FM, de Krijger RR, Eechoute K, Mathijssen RH, et al. Sunitinib-induced hypothyroidism is due to induction of type 3 deiodinase activity and thyroidal capillary regression. Journal of Clinical Endocrinology and Metabolism. 2011;**96**:3087-3094. DOI: 10.1210/jc.2011-1172

[49] Jonklaas J, Bianco AC, Bauer AJ, Burman KD, Cappola AR, Celi FS, et al. Guidelines for the treatment of hypothyroidism: Prepared by the american thyroid association task force on thyroid hormone replacement. Thyroid. 2014;**24**:1670-1751. DOI: 10.1089/thy.2014.0028

[50] Yalcin M, Lin HY, Sudha T, Bharali DJ, Meng R, Tang HY, et al. Response of human pancreatic cancer cell xenografts to tetraiodothyroacetic acid nanoparticles. Hormones & Cancer. 2013;**4**:176-185. DOI: 10.1007/s12672-013-0137-y

[51] Bilen MA, Patel A, Hess KR, Munoz J, Busaidy NL, Wheler JJ, et al. Association between new-onset hypothyroidism and clinical response in patients treated with tyrosine kinase inhibitor therapy in phase I clinical trials. Cancer Chemotherapy and Pharmacology. 2016;**78**:167-171. DOI: 10.1007/s00280-016-3073-z

[52] Hsieh MT, Wang LM, Changou CA, Chin YT, Yang YSH, Lai HY, et al. Crosstalk between integrin αvβ3 and ERα contributes to thyroid hormone-induced proliferation of ovarian cancer cells. Oncotarget. 2017;**8**:24237-24249. DOI: 10.18632/oncotarget.10757

[53] Davis PJ, Hercbergs A, Luidens MK, Lin HY. Recurrence of differentiated thyroid carcinoma during full TSH suppression: Is the tumor now thyroid hormone dependent? Hormones & Cancer. 2015;**6**:7-12. DOI: 10.1007/s12672-014-0204-z

Chapter 2

Bone Tumors: Types and Treatments

Geetanjali B. Tomar, Jay R. Dave, Sayali S. Chandekar and Suhas T. Mhaske

Abstract

The tumors associated with bone are mostly of mesenchymal origin and contribute to approximately 1% of all the known tumors. These could be primary/benign tumors (that originate in the bone), secondary tumors (that originate in some other tissue/organ and metastasize to the bone), or malignant primary bone tumors (that originate in bone and metastasize to distant tissue). These tumors are majorly due to defects in the regulation of tumor suppressor genes and oncogenes and/or misregulation of signal transduction pathways. Chemotherapy and radiotherapy used for the treatment have several side effects. During the recent years, therapeutic strategies involving hormone deprivation (estrogen, androgen), hormone replacements (estrogen analogs), hormone receptor modulators (SERMs), growth factors and cytokines, small-molecule inhibitors, and gene therapy have emerged as a promising alternative to chemo- and radiotherapy. In the present chapter, we have provided an extensive account of tumors associated with the bone and various therapeutic options related to hormone deprivation, hormone replacements, hormone receptor modulators, and hormone inhibition.

Keywords: osteosarcoma, chondrosarcoma, androgen, estrogen, metastasis, hormone

1. Introduction

Primary bone tumors are rare in occurrence accounting for approximately 0.2% of all the tumors. Generally, primary tumors are localized, intra-compartmental, or extended, extra-compartmental [1]. Most benign tumors that have not spread to lymph nodes or other organs remain asymptomatic until their presence is indicated by a trivial insult [1, 2]. Therefore, it becomes important to categorize bone lesions in the early stages of their development for prognosis and diagnosis [2]. On the other hand, skeletal metastases are frequent in patients with breast, prostate, and lung cancer and also occur in other tumors such as myeloma, thyroid and renal cancer, lymphoma, and Ewing's sarcoma [3]. The bone becomes the most common site of metastases in humans due to its highly vascular nature, and this results in pain, pathologic fracture, and decreased quality of life [3].

Bone metastases are either osteolytic or osteoblastic, depending on the dominance of osteoclastic activity or osteoblasts, respectively [3]. As a result the radiological appearance of bone metastasis is lytic, sclerotic, or mixed [4]. General pathogenesis of bone tumors sequentially involves proliferation of primary neoplasm, local tissue invasion, intravasation into blood vessels, extravasation into bone marrow, tumor cell dormancy, proliferation in bone, and modification of bone microenvironment [3]. The site of metastases is governed by the "seed and soil" hypothesis by Paget which states that neoplastic cells grow or proliferate only in a suitable environment [3]. Tumor cells therefore migrate to the heavily vascularized areas of the skeleton, particularly the red bone marrow of the axial skeleton and the proximal ends of the long bones, the ribs, and the vertebral column [5]. Chemotactic factors such as CXCL10 (CXC motif ligand [CXCL]), CXCL12, and osteopontin have been reported to play a major role in tumor migration [6].

Tumors can be classified into low-grade (Grade I), intermediate-grade (Grade II), and high-grade (Grade III) tumors [1]. Grading of bone tumors is roughly based on the cellularity of the lesions compared to the extracellular matrix, nuclear features, the presence of mitotic figures, and necrosis [7]. Grade II tumors are more cellular, with a greater degree of nuclear atypia, hyperchromasia, and nuclear size. Grade III tumors have significant areas of marked pleomorphism, large cells with more hyperchromatic nuclei than Grade II tumors, occasional giant cells, and abundant necrosis [1]. High-grade bone tumors are the fastest growing and most aggressive group of classic osteoblastic subtype. On the basis of histological appearance, bone tumors are classified as parosteal and periosteal. Parosteal tumors belong to low-grade subtype of osteosarcoma, whereas periosteal belongs to the intermediate-grade subtype. Parosteal tumors have fibroblast appearance and are limited to bone surface, but periosteal tumors appear chondroblastic upon histology.

2. Primary malignant tumors

2.1 Giant cell tumor of bone (GCT)

This tumor accounts for 5% of all primary and 20% of the benign skeletal tumors [8]. GCT is an aggressive osteolytic benign bone tumor developing in the long bones, which is characterized by giant, multinucleated osteoclast-like cells, recruited by stromal cells such as osteoblasts [8, 9]. The stromal cells of GCT highly express parathyroid hormone-related peptide (PTHrP) and thus increase the bone tumor cell local invasiveness and migration [9].

Distal femur, proximal tibia, and distal radius are the most common locations for the occurrence of GCT, but due to its association with Paget's disease, it may also occur in the skull, pelvis, facial bones, and spine. It has been reported to rarely affect greater trochanter of the femur. Though some of the reports claim an equal rate of occurrence in both the genders, some reports show an increased prevalence in females [8].

These tumors have been associated with reduction in length of telomeres [7]. Radiological examination in patients with closed physes displays lytic lesions with well-defined, non-sclerotic margins that are eccentric in location and extend near the articular surface. Thus GCT involves cortical expansion or destruction [8].

2.2 Chondrosarcoma

Chondrosarcomas majorly involve tumorous growth of chondrocytes, which are mostly found in bones that elongate due to endochondral ossification and involve differentiation in the epiphyseal growth plates of long bones. For example, hypertrophic chondrocytes are found in clear cell chondrosarcoma. The most common sites include proximal femur, proximal humerus, distal femur, and ribs. Sex hormones such as estrogen play a major role in governing the nuclear signaling pathways involved in this process of ossification [1].

There are different histologic variants of chondrosarcoma.

1. Mesenchymal chondrosarcomas are highly aggressive tumors, composed of resting chondrocytes, and are radiographically and histologically similar to Ewing's sarcoma [1, 10]. Such sarcomas frequently occur in the pelvic bones, femur, and humerus and less commonly in the head, spine, breast, and prostate [1]. These have high risk of local recurrence and distant metastasis [10].

2. Dedifferentiated chondrosarcomas are aggressive neoplasms and have poor prognosis [10].

3. Clear cell chondrosarcomas are low-grade tumors and involve the epiphyseal end of the long bone. The radiographs show a lytic defect at the epiphyseal end of long bones, sharply demarcated with sclerotic margins [10].

4. Extraskeletal myxoid chondrosarcomas are slow-growing tumors, characterized histologically by prominent myxoid degeneration, and are considered as differentiated tumors [10].

5. Juxtacortical chondrosarcoma arises on the surface of the bone and is histologically identical to conventional intramedullary chondrosarcoma [1].

2.3 Ewing's sarcoma

Ewing's sarcoma is an exception to all the bone tumors, because bone tumors are mostly mesenchymal in origin, but Ewing's sarcoma is reported to have neuroectodermal precursor cells [7]. It has been found to be associated with neuroblastomas in patients younger than 5 years, whereas in patients above 30 years, it is associated with small round cell tumors (e.g., small-cell carcinoma) and large-cell lymphoma [1]. Ewing's sarcoma is most likely to occur in younger individuals and most commonly in males [11].

Ewing's sarcoma is characterized by small round cell bone tumor and involves pain at the site of tumor and soft tissue swelling around it [1]. Unlike other primary tumors of the bone, Ewing's sarcoma is associated with a characteristic translocation in the 11th and 22nd chromosomes. This translocation results in production of an aberrant transcription factor EWS/FLI1 that forms a complex with RNA helicase A and drives the pathogenesis of Ewing's sarcoma [7, 11]. Its metastasis involves certain non-specific signs of inflammation, anorexia, fever, malaise, fatigue, and weight loss [1].

2.4 Osteosarcoma

Osteosarcoma is an osteoid-producing malignancy of mesenchymal origin [12]. It is the third most frequent type of cancer in adolescence and represents more than 56% of all bone tumors [13]. It is the most common bone sarcoma and affects 60% of the patients below 25 years of age and 30% of the patients above 40 years [14, 15]. It is associated with extensive genomic disruptions and propensity of metastatic spread. Seventy-six percent of the osteosarcomas have been found to be associated with reduced expression of *HACE1* gene localized to human chromosome 6q21, thus resulting in poor survival [14]. Approximately, 30–40% children with pediatric osteosarcoma die due to metastasis to lungs [1, 16].

Environmental factors such as exposure to radiation, teriparatide (parathyroid hormone 1–34) usage, and consumption of fluorinated drinking water during childhood increase the risk of osteosarcoma [12]. Its localization in regions that are largely cut off from the vasculature reduces the effectiveness of systemically administered chemotherapeutics [17]. The subtypes of osteosarcoma include osteoblastic, chondroblastic, fibroblastic, small cell, telangiectatic, high-grade surface, extraskeletal, and other lower-grade forms of tumors including parosteal and periosteal [12].

Osteosarcomas are one of the widely studied sarcomas of the skeletal system. Several investigations have reported the association of germline mutation disorders such as hereditary retinoblastoma, Rothmund-Thomson syndrome, Li-Fraumeni syndrome, and Bloom syndrome, with increased risk of osteosarcoma [12]. Various other pathways discussed below have been reported to be responsible for supporting growth and metastasis of osteosarcoma.

1. Constitutively active signal transducers and activators of transcription 3 (STAT3) signaling have been found to be necessary for osteosarcoma survival and migration in vitro and tumor growth in vivo. STAT3 is a proto-oncogene that stimulates self-proliferation (due to expression of cyclin D1), mediates immune evasion, promotes angiogenesis, and confers apoptosis resistance (induced by conventional therapies, due to expression of BCL2) [18]. Similarly an upregulation in the expression of survivin (an oncogenic protein) has also been observed in osteosarcoma (**Figure 1**) [19].

2. Attenuation of cell cycle arrest by p53 has been found to affect the upstream p53 signaling pathways [20]. Approximately 26.5% of non-hereditary osteosarcomas have been reported to be associated with somatic loss of p53, out of which 60% are high-grade osteosarcomas, whereas 1% are low-grade osteosarcomas [14]. Tumor suppressor genes such as p15 and p27 have been commonly found to be silenced due to methylation of promoter by DNA methyl transferase that adds methyl group to the fifth carbon position of cytosine ring in CpG islands, leading to heterochromatin and inhibition of gene expression (**Figure 1**) [21].

3. Sex steroid hormones have been found to play an important role in development and progression of bone tumors. Previous investigations have revealed the role of aromatase and sulfatase pathways in the in situ formation of active estrogen. Aromatase pathway involves aromatization of androgens to produce estrogen. In sulfatase pathway, estrone 3-sulfate is taken up by the cells and is activated by the removal of sulfate by steroid sulfatase, thus converting inactive estrogen to unconjugated and bioactive estrogen. Both these pathways allow generation of estrogen and androgen by the bone cells in the bone microenvironment (**Figure 2**) [24].

4. Growth factors such as transforming growth factor (TGF)-β, insulin-like growth factors (IGFs), bone morphogenetic proteins (BMPs), platelet-derived growth factor (PDGF), and fibroblast growth factor (FGF) released from degraded bone matrices also promote tumor cell proliferation by production of PTHrP that interacts with parathyroid hormone (PTH)/PTHrP receptors in the bone and kidney to cause hypercalcemia, osteoclast-mediated bone resorption, increased nephrogenous cyclic AMP, and phosphate excretion [4–6, 25]. PTH is known to regulate osteosarcoma cells, by inducing transcription of c-Fos that in turn targets calcium/cAMP-response element (CRE) through activation of protein kinase A (PKA) [26]. c-Fos is a member of activator protein-1 (AP-1) family of transcription factors containing c-Fos (FosB, Fra-1, Fra-2) (**Figure 1**) [27].

Additionally, FGF also regulates multiple signaling cascades in both autocrine and paracrine manner [4]. FGF receptor 1 was identified as a c-Fos-regulated gene playing an important role in lung metastases of osteosarcoma. The FGF receptors 1–4 belong to a family of receptor tyrosine kinase (RTK) that triggers intracellular signaling cascades through mitogen-activated protein kinase (MAPK), phosphoinositide 3-kinase (PI3K)/protein kinase B (AKT), STAT pathways, and signal transducers phospholipase Cγ (PLCγ) and casitas B-lineage lymphoma (CBL) (**Figure 1**) [27].

5. Majority of the osteosarcomas develop as a result of metastases of breast, prostate, or lung tumors into the bone. Breast cancer cells metastasize to the bone and secrete various factors in the bone microenvironment that enhance osteoclastogenesis and inhibit osteoblastogenesis, thus developing several skeletal-related events (SREs) such as pathological fracture, spinal cord compression, bone pain, and hypercalcemia [28]. Similarly, androgen signaling components such as androgen receptor, ARV7, v-ets avian erythroblastosis virus E26 oncogene homolog (ERG), cytochrome P450, and family 17 subfamily A polypeptide 1 (CYP17) and molecules such as phospho-Met, phospho-Src, glucocorticoid receptor, and Ki67 have been implicated to play a major role in the metastasis of castration-resistant prostate cancer (CRPC) [29].

Some of the reports associate migration and invasion of breast cancer cells to the upregulation of micro RNAs, miR-10b, miR-373, and miR-520c. Out of these, miR-373 and miR-520c have been found to silence *CD44* gene that codes for hyaluronan receptor (plays an important in cellular adhesion). Similarly, miR-218 that is involved in osteoblast differentiation promotes breast cancer cell osteomimicry (ability to acquire bone cell phenotype for immune escape). miR-154 and miR-379 overexpression in bone metastatic cells was associated with mesenchymal properties and enhanced invasive potential [30].

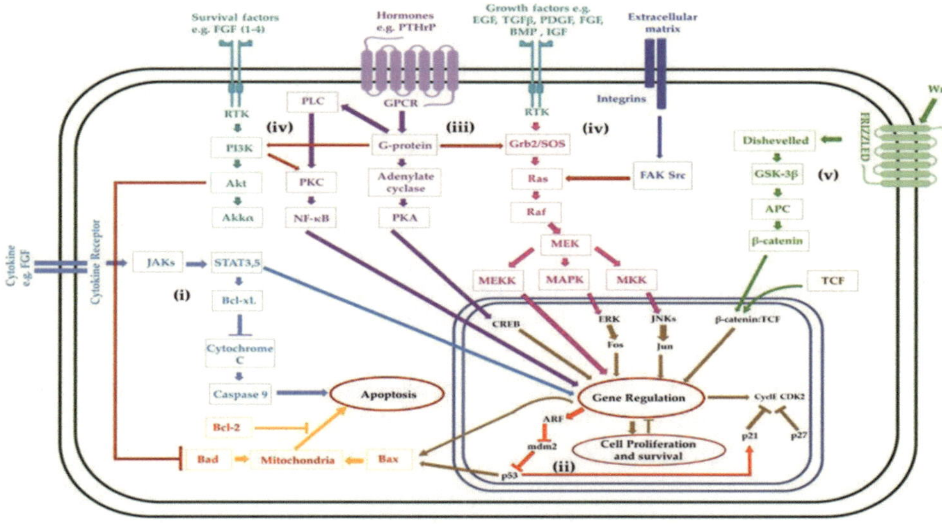

Figure 1.
Cross talk of various signaling pathways in osteosarcoma. (i) JAK–STAT pathway confers apoptosis resistance, thus enhancing tumor cell survival. (ii) Inactivation of p53 favors cell cycle progression in cells with DNA damage and promotes tumorigenesis. (iii) Cross talk between GPCR-regulated PTHrP signaling and RTK-mediated survival/growth factors. (iv) Role of RTK in supporting tumor cell survival and proliferation as a response to various growth factors. (v) Wnt signaling mechanism plays a major role in tumors associated with bone tissue.

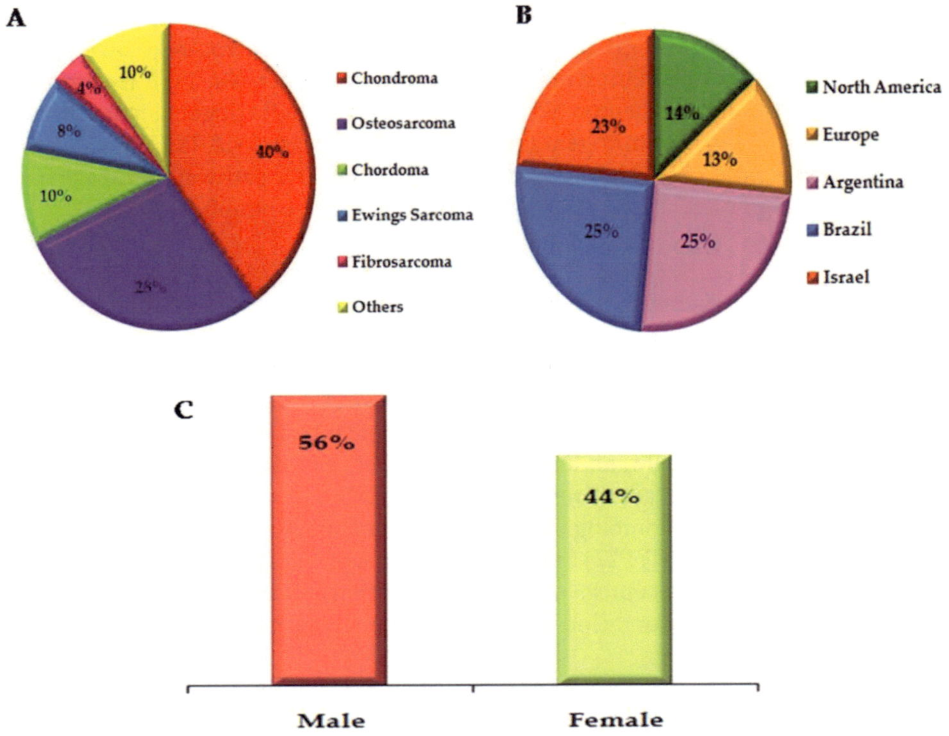

Figure 2.
(A) Percentage of primary bone cancers in adult human population [22]. (B) Osteosarcoma cases per 100,000 population per year [23]. (C) Percentage of males and females diagnosed with primary bone tumor in the United States in the year 2017 [22].

3. Pathophysiology of bone tumors

General pathogenesis of bone tumors sequentially involves proliferation of primary neoplasm, local tissue invasion, intravasation into blood vessels, extravasation into bone marrow, tumor cell dormancy, proliferation in the bone, and modification of bone microenvironment. The site of metastases is governed by the "seed and soil" hypothesis by Paget which states that neoplastic cells grow or proliferate only in a suitable environment [3].

The initial step in metastasis involves escape of cancer cells from primary tumor into the systemic circulation, through epithelial–mesenchymal transition (EMT). EMT involves loss of cell surface intercellular adhesion proteins and epithelial polarization. EMT is followed by dissolution of the extracellular matrix by secreting certain proteolytic enzymes and migration into surrounding tissue to enter systemic circulation through intravasation. Such circulating tumor cells (CTCs) escape anoikis (cell apoptosis due to loss of cell-matrix or cell-cell interactions, preferably through overexpression of tyrosine kinase receptor, TrkB) resulting in activation of PI3K-AKT pro-survival pathways. These tumor cells also upregulate certain proteins on their surface (e.g., CD47) to escape destruction by macrophages [4]. The two major factors that govern the localization of CTCs are blood flow and molecular signaling. For example, the metastasis of breast cancer to thoracic spine is due to the venous drainage of the breast to thoracic region, whereas lung cancer shows general skeletal distribution due to the drainage of pulmonary veins into the left side of the heart, followed by eventual entry into systemic circulation. Alternatively, prostate cancer majorly displays metastasis to the axial skeletal in the lumbar spine, sacrum, and pelvis due to their drainage through pelvic plexus. As far as the signaling pathways are concerned, CXCL12-CXCR4 (CXC motif ligand [CXCL], CXC chemokine receptor [CXCR]) axis has been found to regulate CTC homing to the bone. CXCL12, also called as stromal cell-derived factor 1 (SDF1), is a chemokine factor secreted by bone marrow MSCs, endothelial cells, and osteoblast and primarily binds to G protein-coupled receptor, CXCR4, thus activating cell survival, chemotaxis, and expression of integrin $\alpha v\beta 3$ on the surface of CTCs [4]. Another receptor involved in osteotropism is the calcium-sensing receptor (CaSR), expressed by advanced primary breast tumors that causes enhanced calcium-induced migration to the bone [30]. In addition to CXCL12-CXCR4 axis, non-receptor cytoplasmic tyrosine kinase, Src, has also been shown to mediate improved survival of breast cancer cells in the bone marrow by increasing the resistance to tumor necrosis factor (TNF)-related apoptosis-inducing ligand (TRAIL) and activation of AKT signaling [4].

After tumor cells colonize the bone, they induce the expression of receptor activator of nuclear factor-κB ligand (RANKL) via production of PTHrP, prostaglandin E2 (PGE2), interleukin 6 (IL-6), IL-1β, TNF, and epidermal growth factor (EGF), which promote osteoclast differentiation and activation. RANKL induces osteoclastic bone resorption resulting in growth of osteolytic tumor that causes hypercalcemia, and it also acts as a chemoattractant to the bone for tumor cells [6]. In relation to this, hypoxia-inducible factor (HIF)-1α has been reported to act as an upstream master switch to many of the osteolytic factors such as IL-11 and IL-8 and angiogenic factors such as PDGF and vascular endothelial growth factor (VEGF) [4, 31]. TGF-β plays a central role in the pathogenesis of osteolytic bone metastasis from breast carcinoma via potentiation of estrogen receptor (ER)-α-mediated transcription induced by constitutively active ERα [25]. A higher expression of ERα in the cortical bone suggests its role in bone formation, whereas trabecular bone cells show a higher expression of ERβ [32].

Osteolytic bone metastases are most often caused by breast cancer and multiple myeloma [6, 33], whereas osteoblastic metastases are mostly observed in bone metastasis of prostate cancer, which is due to osteoblast stimulation by cancer cells [6, 34]. Factors that are locally produced by cancer cells, such as bone BMP, IGF, FGF, TGF-β, and endothelin-1, also promote osteoblast proliferation and bone formation [6].

Another important cellular component of bone microenvironment that is involved in tumor metastases is osteocytes. Osteocytes present in the bone regulate osteoclast development through expression of RANKL, macrophage colony-stimulating factor (M-CSF), and osteoprotegerin (OPG) and inhibit osteoblast differentiation by the expression of sclerostin. Osteocytes have an interesting ability to respond to mechanical stress and pressure. An increase in pressure due to prostate cancer metastasis thus results in upregulation of matrix metalloproteinases (MMPs) and chemokine (C-C motif) ligand 5 (CCL-5). Additionally, apoptotic osteocytes have been shown to release IL-11 that enhances osteoclast differentiation. Endothelial cells are yet another important component of the bone marrow that contributes to the bone metastatic process. Endothelial cells in the metaphysis of the long bone aid CTC adhesion due to constitutive expression of P-selectin, E-selectin, vascular cell adhesion molecule 1 (VCAM1), and intercellular adhesion molecule A (ICAM-1). Decrease in shear forces due to reduced blood flow velocity in the large volume of sinusoids also favors CTC attachment [4].

The bone marrow is also a major reservoir for dendritic cells, macrophages, myeloid-derived cells, and different subsets of T cells. T and B cells are known to produce RANKL and impact osteoclastogenesis, whereas production of IL-6, IL-23, and IL-1 by dendritic cells in the bone microenvironment of multiple myeloma patients causes an increase in Th17 cells that in turn increase IL-17. IL-17 is an important cytokine that promotes osteoclast and myeloma proliferation and also mediates interactions between T cells and bone metastatic environment. Additionally, myeloid-derived suppressor cells from the bone marrow suppress innate and adaptive immune responses by impairing T-cell antigen recognition and promotion of regulatory T cells [4].

However, as an individual ages, the hematopoietic red bone marrow gets converted to adipose tissue-rich yellow bone marrow that has a significant impact on the development of bone metastasis. These bone marrow adipocytes not only serve as an energy source but also secrete several pro-inflammatory mediators such as IL-1β, IL-6, leptin, adiponectin, VCAM-1, TNF-α, and CXCL12 that increase cancer cell survival and proliferation [4].

4. Tumor biomarkers

Histological examination of tissue biopsy has been the most commonly used procedure for the diagnosis of bone tumors. Clinical and radiological observations also aid in diagnosis and provide a complete staging of bone cancers. But molecular and genetic markers increase the accuracy of diagnosis, assist in subtyping bone tumors, and also provide an overview of target molecules for designing therapeutic approaches. The biomarkers can be specific or non-specific; diagnostic, prognostic, or therapeutic; and serological, genetic, or histological. The clinical presentation of bone tumors is non-specific, and the most common symptoms include pain and swelling. The clinical features involve limited movement, skin hyperthermia, weight loss, and the presence of a visible mass in the anatomical profile [10].

The serological markers are generally a reflection of osteoblastic and osteoclastic activities in the bone [10]. As mentioned in the earlier sections, breast cancer metastases are mostly osteolytic, whereas metastases of prostate cancer are generally osteoblastic. Therefore, elevated levels of urinary N-terminal cross-linked telopeptide (NTx of type I collagen) and serum carboxyterminal cross-linked telopeptide (ICTP of type I collagen) in solid tumor patients and serum tartrate-resistant acid phosphatase type 5b (TRAcP-5b) in patients with breast tumor metastasis can be used for diagnosis. On the other hand, serum levels of bone-specific alkaline phosphatase (BSAP), procollagen type I N-terminal propeptide (PINP), and OPG serve as the biomarkers for prostate cancer metastasis [10, 30].

With reference to the genetic changes, sarcomas can be divided into three categories: sarcomas with specific translocations (e.g., Ewing's sarcoma, aneurysmal bone cyst), tumors with gene mutations or amplifications (e.g., chondrosarcomas, fibrous dysplasia), and sarcomas with genetic instability. These cytogenetic changes can be detected using banding and multicolor fluorescence in situ hybridization (FISH), array comparative genomic hybridization (array CGH), targeted detection techniques such as qPCR, and techniques to detect mutation [10].

There are several markers that are used for prognosis or diagnosis of different types of tumors that are discussed below:

4.1 Osteosarcoma

4.1.1 Serum markers

1. Degradation of collagen and the ground substance in the bone (due to prolonged exposure to fluoride) results in increased concentration of serum sialic acid that can be used as a serum biomarker for osteosarcoma [10].

2. Expression of heat shock protein (HSP gp96), in the cytoplasm of osteoblastic sarcoma, has been found to be associated with pathogenesis of bone tumors. But it does not provide any idea regarding the degree of malignancy [10].

3. The osteosarcoma patients displayed increased levels of endostatin, placental growth factor (PlGF), and FGF-1 and FGF-2 in serum [10].

4. Gas chromatography–mass spectrometry profiles of small-molecule metabolites in urine and serum samples of osteosarcoma patients displayed a disrupted energy metabolism, downregulated amino acid metabolism, and increase in glutathione metabolism and polyamine metabolism [10].

5. qPCR and western blot analysis for detection of IGF-1 receptor showed its increased expression in osteosarcoma tissues, suggesting it as a prognostic marker. Western blotting and enzyme-linked immunosorbent assay (ELISA) confirmed a decrease in serum levels of gelsolin in the osteosarcoma samples [10].

6. The presence of FGF-2 or leukemia inhibitory factor (Lif) serves as a biomarker, suggesting reduction of osteogenesis on osteosarcoma cells. Elevated serum levels of CXCL4 and CXCL in osteosarcoma patients affirmed the role of these markers in clinical manifestation. In addition to this, biomarker Snail2 is also useful in prognosis of bone tumors [10].

7. Metastatic prostate cancers have been found to express the well-known markers of aggressiveness, namely, prostatic-specific antigen (PSA) [30].

8. Increase in erythrocyte sedimentation rate (ESR), alkaline phosphatase (ALP), and lactate dehydrogenase (LDH) are indicators of osteosarcoma [1, 12].

9. Immunohistochemistry of primary osteosarcomas showed expression of mitotic arrest defective protein 2 (MAD2). Immunohistochemical analysis of osteosarcoma biopsies indicated reduced expression of cysteine-rich protein with Kazal motifs (RECK). Immunohistochemistry analysis also showed expression of WNT-5a and ROR2 in patients with advanced stages of osteosarcoma [10].

4.1.2 Genetic markers

Assessment of *CCN3* expression levels at diagnosis may represent a useful molecular tool for early identification of patients with osteosarcoma. Gene alteration of c-kit protein also serves as a prognostic marker for osteosarcoma. The transcriptional regulator, Oct-4, has been found to play a marked role in proliferation and spread of cancer. A reduced expression and inactivation of miR-34 gene have been reported to be associated with osteosarcomas. The action of miR-34 is p53 dependent. A dominant polymorphic variant of TGFβ receptor 1 (TGFBR1), TGFBR1*6A, is found to be associated with increased susceptibility of osteosarcoma for metastasis. Bcl-xL, a member of Bcl-2 (B-cell lymphoma (BCL)) protein family, has been investigated to function as a dominant regulator of apoptotic cell death and plays an important role in malignant transformation. Cytotoxic T-lymphocyte antigen-4 (CTLA-4), a molecule that decreases immune response mediated by T cells, promotes development of osteosarcoma. Overexpressions of *Cortactin* (*CTTN*) gene, present in 11q13 amplicon, serve as a valid biomarker for osteosarcoma [10].

4.2 Ewing's sarcoma

Ewing's sarcomas are associated with rearrangement of the *EWS* gene on chromosome 22q12 with an erythroblast transformation-specific (*ETS*) gene family member, resulting in formation of EWS-ETS fusion protein (EWS-FLI). FLI1 has been suggested as a useful marker particularly when hematolymphoid markers are negative. This translocation defines Ewing's sarcoma family of tumors (ESFT) and provides a major tool for their accurate diagnosis. The translocation results in different types of genetic abnormalities, e.g., five forms of EWSR1-FLI1, three forms of EWSR1-ERG, and one form of EWSR1-FEV. A high expression of BMI-1 in ESFT cells was found to significantly affect survival and proliferation. Expression of CXCR4 has been reported to increase the risk of tumor metastases, whereas CXCR7 expression is associated with shorter survival [10].

Ewing's sarcoma has been reported to be associated with modulation of RANKL by VEGF-165, thus resulting in activation of osteoclast-mediated bone destruction [10].

4.3 Chondrosarcoma

On the basis of histological observations, chondrosarcomas are classified into three categories:

Grade I (low grade)—cytology similar to enchondroma and hyperchromatic plump nuclei of uniform size [10].

Grade II (intermediate grade)—increased cellularity, hyperchromasia, distinct nucleoli, and foci of myxoid alteration [10].

Grade III (high grade)—increased cellularity and nuclear atypia, occasional giant cells, abundant necrosis, and presence of mitosis [10].

4.3.1 Genetic markers

Deletions in the loci of *CDKN2A*, *EXT1*, and *EXT2* genes, *p53* mutation as late event in tumor progression, and amplification of 12q13 and loss of 9p21 are genetic aberrations found in conventional chondrosarcomas [10].

Higher expression of PTHR1 and Bcl-2 was found to be associated with increasing histological grade in chondrosarcoma, suggesting its involvement in tumor progression. A higher expression of Aurora kinases A and B was relevant as prognosis marker for chondrosarcoma. Somatic heterozygous isocitrate dehydrogenase 1 (IDH1) hot spots (R132C and R132H) or IDH2 (R172S) mutations are specifically found in cartilaginous tumors [10].

4.3.2 Biological and molecular markers

qPCR analysis showed a high expression of COX-2 protein in solitary peripheral chondrosarcoma. Some of the studies reported a significant role of nitrotyrosine, COX-2, CD34, and lymphatic marker podoplanin with histological grades of chondrosarcoma. Molecules such as integrin-linked kinase α and β-parvin and Mig-2 allow attachment of cells to matrix and govern cell motility and growth, thus playing an important role in progression and prognosis of chondrosarcomas [10].

Significantly high serum levels of receptor activator of nuclear factor-κB (RANK), OPG, IL-8, IL-6, and OPG/soluble RANKL ratio have been used to detect bone tumors. Osteosarcoma patients display a higher serum concentration of IL-16 as compared to chondrosarcoma patients [35].

5. Diagnosis

1. **Radiographic diagnosis**: Plain radiographs, computed tomography (CT) scans, and magnetic resonance imaging (MRI) are used to investigate the extent of tumors and to study the surrounding structure such as blood vessels, nerves, and soft tissues [1, 12].

2. **Positron emission tomography (PET)-CT**: [F-18]-Fluorodeoxy-D-glucose (FDG)-PET is a noninvasive imaging tool used for accurate discrimination between responding and nonresponding osseous tumors [1, 12].

3. **Bone scintigraphy**: This method involves total body scan and identifies axial and appendicular skeletal metastasis. It helps in determining intraosseous extension of tumors and sites of metastasis [1, 12].

4. **Thallium scintigraphy**: This method is used for determining tumor response to neoadjuvant (preoperative) chemotherapy when MRI is not helpful and also for detection of local recurrence [1].

5. **Incisional or core needle biopsy** is the final step in the diagnostic process. The tumor is staged using the Musculoskeletal Tumor Society staging scheme or the American Joint Commission on Cancer (AJCC) system [12].

6. **Increased uptake of technetium diphosphonate** in the clinical bone scans of osteolytic lesions in cancer patients also provides a diagnostic tool to identify increased cellular activity and metastasis [36].

Bone scans, X-rays, and histologic evaluation of autopsy specimens are commonly used for radiologic and histologic assessment of tumor sites [5].

6. Therapy

Osteosarcoma is typically treated with surgery and adjuvant chemotherapy that usually includes a combination of methotrexate, doxorubicin, and cisplatin [37]. Once the cancer has spread to the bones, it can rarely be cured, but often it can be treated to slow down its growth [38]. The therapeutic strategies for bone tumors should involve the following:

1. Treatment of cancer cells: This involves inhibition of tumor cell proliferation or killing of cancer cells to extend the patient's survival time. This could be achieved by usage of cytotoxic drugs, hormonal deprivation, or inhibition of specific signaling pathways by targeted agents [4].

2. Disruption of the vicious cycle created due to complex biological signaling between cancer cells and bone resident cells [4].

3. Palliative therapies to reduce the extremely debilitating and painful symptom of bone metastasis and improve the quality of life for cancer patients [4].

As discussed in the previous sections, various signaling pathway are involved in the proliferation and migration of tumor cells. Targeting these signaling pathways by use of different inhibitors could hamper the survival of tumor cells. However, it has already been known that the sex hormones play a major role in tumor cell survival and metastases. Thus, hormone therapy for curing tumors would basically involve hormone deprivation approaches. These strategies might inhibit the action of hormones responsible to bone metastases, resulting in osteolytic or osteoblastic tumors.

6.1 Androgen deprivation therapy (ADT)

Ubiquitous and extensive expression of androgen receptor in the bone marrow of both males and females of all ages provides a direct evidence of action of androgen on the bone marrow and offers clues to clinicopathological correlates [39]. Most prostate cancers and their stages depend upon androgen and androgen receptor (AR) for their growth and survival. Androgen receptor is a transcription factor that regulates the expression of several genes in response to binding of androgen (such as testosterone and dihydrotestosterone) and thus regulates the process of proliferation and survival. As mentioned earlier, bone metastasis of prostate cancers majorly results in osteoblastic bone tumors [40]. Therefore, systemic treatment for advanced prostate cancer involves androgen deprivation therapy (ADT) that includes the following approaches:

a. To reduce the levels of circulating androgen by surgical or chemical castration. Surgical castration results in reduction of circulating androgen levels by >90% within 24 hours, whereas chemical castration is achieved by application of analogs of luteinizing hormone-releasing hormone (LH-RH) and results in reduction of circulating levels of testosterone [40].

LH-RH is a neurohormone, secreted by the hypothalamus, and regulates the secretion of gonadotropin, luteinizing hormone (LH), and follicle-stimulating hormone (FSH) from the pituitary. LH-RH acts via binding to its receptor, LH-RHR. These receptors have also been found in the cytoplasm of many tumor cells that involve both reproductive and nonreproductive tissues. LH-RH agonists and antagonists have been found to downregulate these receptors and thus inhibit tumor growth [41]. Leuprolide acetate (Lupron, Eligard), goserelin acetate (Zoladex), triptorelin (Trelstar), and histrelin (Vantas) are some of the LH-RH agonists, whereas degarelix is an antagonist [4, 40]. LH-RHR can also be targeted specifically by peptides conjugated to anticancer drugs, thus developing cytotoxic analogs [41]. AN-152, commercially designated as AEZS-108, has been developed by conjugating 14-OH group of doxorubicin (DOX) to epsilon-amino group of D-Lys side chain of carrier peptide, through a glutaric acid spacer. The drug is endocytosed by cells through receptor-mediated endocytosis and thus selectively acts on cells that express its receptor. After internalization the drug is cleaved from the LH-RH moiety and accumulates in the nucleus. Because of receptor-mediated entry, the drug shows lesser side effects and also overcomes the resistance [41].

Administration of LH-RH agonist or antagonist for ADT not only results in suppression of testosterone to castration levels but also depletes estradiol, because it is derived by aromatization of testosterone [42]. Estradiol deficiency negatively impacts the bone health resulting in decline of bone mineral density (BMD) and increased risk of fractures [42]. This decrease in bone density also results in development of renal stones leading to risk of urinary calculi [43]. Recently parenteral (e.g., intravenous, intramuscular, or transdermal) administration of estradiol has been investigated to suppress androgen production through negative feedback loop involving hypothalamic–pituitary axis and avoids fall in endogenous estradiol levels. This also eliminates the risk of embolic cardiovascular toxicity that was caused due to oral administration of estradiol [42].

b. To prevent binding of androgen to AR, by competitive inhibition using antiandrogens. These molecules compete with androgen for the ligand-binding domain of AR [40]. The antiandrogens can be of two categories, steroidal and nonsteroidal. Cyproterone acetate, a derivative of hydroxyprogesterone, is a steroidal antiandrogen and an antigonadotropin, which has a binding affinity for AR. But it has been found that it is not a pure antagonist but rather a partial agonist that adversely affects the survival of prostate cancer patients when combined with castration [40]. Among the nonsteroidal antiandrogens are the first-generation flutamide, nilutamide, and bicalutamide and second-generation enzalutamide and the cytochrome P450 c17 (CYP17, a critical enzyme in testosterone synthesis) inhibitor, abiraterone acetate, which prevents synthesis of androgens. Abiraterone inhibits 17-α-hydroxylase/17,20 lyase, a testosterone synthesis enzyme found in the adrenals, testis, and tumor [40, 44]. All these nonsteroidal antiandrogens are similar in terms of the chemical structure of their moiety that binds to the ligand-binding pocket [40]. It has been found that treatment with abiraterone acetate plus prednisone prolongs survival among patients with metastatic castration-resistant prostate cancer [44], though back pain, nausea, constipation, bone pain, arthralgia, urinary tract infection, edema, cardiac events, and elevation in levels of aminotransferase are some of the side effects associated with administration of abiraterone [44, 45].

Flutamide was the first nonsteroidal antiandrogen drug approved by the US Food and Drug Administration (FDA) for prostate cancer and forms the basis for all other nonsteroidal antiandrogens. The recommended dose of flutamide is 250 mg three times per day, so as to achieve a Cmax and Cmin of approximately 1.7 and 0.8 μg/ml, respectively. It acts via blocking the binding of androgen to the ligand-binding pocket of AR, resulting in inhibition of nuclear translocation of androgen-bound AR. But improvement in disease upon cessation of flutamide treatment has been observed in patients, due to gain-of-function mutation in the ligand-binding domain of AR, T877A. Flutamide gets eliminated through the kidney, and liver toxicity is one of the common adverse effects [40].

Enzalutamide (previously called MDV3100) also acts via inhibiting the binding of androgen to AR, thus blocking its nuclear translocation and interaction with co-activators [4, 29, 40, 46]. Its recommended dose is 160 mg/day [40, 47]. However, clinical resistance due to gain-of-function mutation in AR ligand-binding domain (F876 L) and constitutive expression of active spice variants of AR that lack ligand-binding domain results in poor survival rates. Apalutamide and darolutamide also belong to the second generation of nonsteroidal antiandrogen that blocks the androgen binding to AR [40].

A novel first class of drug, ralaniten, is currently under clinical trials for patients who have previously received abiraterone, enzalutamide, or both. This class of drug binds to the unique region in the N-terminal domain of both full-length and truncated constitutively active splice variant of AR [40].

c. ADT that effectively reduces the serum testosterone levels has been a core tool for treating metastatic and advanced prostate cancer [48]. However, neoadjuvant ADT has been suggested to have several advantages in prostate cancer patients undergoing transperineal prostate brachytherapy. The agents that are mainly used as adjuvant ADT include estrogens, antiandrogen monotherapy, and combined androgen blockade (CAB) using antiandrogen plus a gonadotropin-releasing hormone receptor (GnRH) agonist. It has been reported that in comparison to GnRH agonist, degarelix, a GnRH receptor antagonist, is more efficient in achieving castration levels of testosterone and PSA, without risk of testosterone flare [48, 49].

ADT is the mainstay of treatment for advanced prostate cancer, but eventual development of castration-resistant prostate cancer (CRPC) reduces the survival rates. One of the main reasons for development of CRPC is the sustained levels of androgen within the tumor due to suboptimal androgen suppression by primary ADT. Moreover, apart from the hormone-independent subsets, the other subsets of CRPC cells adapt themselves to the low testosterone environment induced by ADT and become hypersensitive to even lower concentrations of testosterone and other androgen precursors. Therefore, secondary hormone therapies are proving to be more efficient to achieve maximum suppression of testosterone. GTx-758 (3-fluoro-N-(4-fluorophenyl)-4-hydroxy-N-(4-hydroxyphenyl) benzamide) is an oral nonsteroidal selective estrogen receptor (ERα) agonist that lowers the free testosterone and PSA levels by increasing sex hormone-binding globulin (SHBG). This also helps to avoid side effects related to estrogen deficiency [50].

Finasteride and dutasteride (5α-reductase enzyme inhibitors) are found to inhibit 5α-reductase-mediated conversion of testosterone to the high affinity androgen receptor ligand, 5α-dihydrotestosterone [51].

6.2 Selective estrogen receptor modulators (SERMs)

Estrogen is chemically related compounds derived from androgen precursors but contain a defining aromatic and hydroxyl group at the 17th position. Estrogens comprise the natural ligands for estrogen receptors (ERs), with 17β-estradiol being a potent agonist. 17β-estradiol has been reported to inhibit metastasis-associated lung adenocarcinoma transcript 1 (MALAT-1)-mediated osteosarcoma migration, invasion, metastasis, and induction of cell apoptosis, in an estrogen receptor α (ERα)-independent manner [15]. Earlier it was thought that binding of ER agonists induces a conformational change in the receptors, conferring the ability for co-activators to bind, whereas ER antagonists were thought to compete for binding [52]. But later studies with tamoxifen revealed that the same molecule can behave as an agonist (tamoxifen acts as an estrogen agonist in the uterus, promoting hypertrophy) as well as an antagonist (tamoxifen exhibited estrogenic activity in the bone, thus protecting against bone loss), depending on the tissue context. Recently it has been found that oxysterols such as 27-hydroxycholesterol (27 HC) also modulate the activity of estrogen receptors (ERs) and are therefore classified as endogenous SERMs. 27 HC is derived from cholesterol in the presence of enzyme CYP27A1 (cytochrome P450 enzyme). Breast cancer is the most common cancer in women, and its metastasis is majorly hormone (estrogen receptor) dependent. Some of the reports emphasize on the role of 27 HC in cancer progression and drug resistance, but several other reports also highlight its beneficial role in inhibiting proliferation and invasion of prostate cancer cells by blocking sterol-regulatory element-binding protein 2 (SREBP2). However, their different affinities for the different subtypes of ERs (α and β) and different relative expressions of these subtypes in tissues may explain some the of SERMs' pharmacology. Recent evidence also suggests that binding of the receptor even by structurally related compounds could result in unique conformational changes, thus allowing recruitment of distinct sets of co-activators and/or corepressors to the receptor [52].

SERMs such as genistein, daidzein, and 4-hydroxytamoxifen have been reported to downregulate the expression of epidermal growth factor (EGFR) in vitro in osteosarcoma cells in an ER-dependent manner. The reduction in EGFR expression resulted in upregulation of markers for osteoblast differentiation, thus resulting in suppression of tumor cell proliferation [53].

Isoflavones such as genistein and daidzein are abundantly found in soybeans and soy-based food products. Isoflavones, coumestans, and lignans belong to a class of phytoestrogens. Phytoestrogens are plant-derived substances that resemble 17β-estradiol and can bind to activate intracellular estrogen receptors. These dietary phytoestrogens have been reported to exhibit bone-protecting effect without the risk of breast cancer [54].

Genistein has also been demonstrated to elicit different cell responses through different signaling mechanisms. A combination of genistein and 17β-estradiol has been shown to significantly increase apoptosis of breast cancer cells by increasing the BAX/BCL-2 (BCL-2-associated X protein (BAX)) ratio and reducing phosphorylation of extracellular signal-regulated kinase (ERK) ½ and AKT [55].

6.3 Activation of ERα

Osteosarcoma is a malignant tumor in the bone that originates from osteoblasts or osteoblast precursors. The reports clarify that normal osteoblasts express ERα, whereas osteosarcomas do not (due to promoter DNA methylation). Thus a treatment strategy that involves induction of ERα expression in osteosarcoma cells in combination with estrogen administration would reduce proliferation of osteosarcoma and increase cell differentiation. In vitro treatment of osteosarcoma cells with decitabine (DAC, 5-Aza-2′-deoxycytidine) has been found to induce the expression of ERα but reduce the expression of metastasis-associated markers such as vimentin, slug, zeb1, and MMP9, with simultaneous decrease in stem cell markers such as *SOX2*, *OCT4*, and *NANOG*. Subsequent treatment with 17β-estradiol synergized with DAC in reducing cell proliferation and inducing differentiation markers such as alkaline phosphatase, osterix, and bone sialoproteins [21].

6.4 Estrogen inhibitors

The bone is the frequent site for metastasis of breast cancer. Estrogen plays a critical role in development and progression of breast cancer by interacting with ERα and ERβ. In postmenopausal women, estrogens (estrone and estradiol) are synthesized from androgens (androstenedione and testosterone) at extragonadal sites, including the breast. Thus the third generation of therapy involves inhibition of these aromatase enzymes, catalyzing the conversion of androgens to estrogens [56]. The aromatase inhibitors fall into two categories: steroidal and nonsteroidal. Letrozole and anastrozole are the third-generation nonsteroidal aromatase inhibitors that block the extragonadal conversion of androgens to estrogens and give rise to an estrogen-depleted environment [51, 56, 57]. This lowers the estrogen in breast tissues and reduces their metastasis to the bone [56]. But in patients with hormone receptor-positive breast cancer, both the disease and its therapeutic treatment with antiestrogenic agents negatively impact the bone and result in decrease in bone mineral density. Therefore anti-hormonal therapy is considered only in cases where cancer cells express the ERα [58]. However, unlike nonsteroidal aromatase inhibitors, a steroidal aromatase inhibitor, e.g., exemestane (probably due to its steroid structure), has been reported to exert beneficial effects on the bone through its primary metabolite 17-hydroexemestane [51, 57].

Fulvestrant, an alkylosulfonian derivative of estradiol, is another category of estrogen inhibitors (estrogen receptor antagonist), which competitively binds to ER with high affinity and downregulates expression of ERβ by functional blockade [59, 60]. Fulvestrant has been reported to induce mitochondrial depolarization at high concentrations that results in release of apoptogenic factors, loss of oxidative phosphorylation, and eventually cell death due to apoptosis [60].

2-Methoxyestradiol (2-ME) belongs to another class of anticancer drugs, which act via induction of neuronal nitric oxide synthase and generation of nitric oxide in the nuclei of cancer cells. However, recently 2-ME has been found to activate epigenetically silenced ERβ, resulting in apoptosis of malignant cancer cells [60].

Furthermore, some of the recent reports emphasize the role of mutant ERα gene (*ESR1*) in cancer progression and drug resistance. These mutations have been observed to get accumulated in circulating DNA of bone metastasis patients [32].

6.5 Estrogen replacement

Zoledronic acid is a known anti-resorptive agent and exhibits antitumor effects in ER-ve breast cancers. Some of the recent studies emphasize that it's the menopausal status (and not the hormone receptor status) that determines its anticancer efficiency [61]. This differential effect of zoledronic acid in pre- and postmenopausal bone metastasis patients has been suggested to be regulated by bone turnover effect of estrogen. Estrogen inhibits osteoclastogenesis via its direct effect on osteoclast and their precursors. Similarly, zoledronic acid also exhibits pro-apoptotic effects on osteoclasts by inhibiting mevalonate pathway and thus prevents release of growth factors that stimulate tumor growth. But in contrast to estrogen, zoledronic acid also reduces the number and activity of osteoblasts. Therefore, replacement of estrogen with zoledronic acid could be a more effective antitumor therapy in a low-estrogen bone microenvironment. Though administration of zoledronic acid does not alter growth of ER+ve cells at the primary site of tumor, it hampers their dissemination in the bone. As the cells evade the bone microenvironment, zoledronic acid-mediated bone turnover inhibits their proliferation and prevents overt metastases. Thus zoledronic acid could inhibit bone metastases of both ER-ve and ER+ve breast cancer cells [61].

One of the study reports dealing with in vitro microarray data analysis revealed that glucocorticoid was more efficient in controlling osteosarcoma cell growth than 17β estradiol. Glucocorticoid upregulated the expression of tumor suppressor genes resulting in apoptosis and downregulated the oncogenes associated with cell cycle and mitosis, whereas estradiol had an opposite action [62].

7. Conclusion

Primary bone tumors are a rare occurrence, and most of the bone tumors arise due to metastases of breast, prostate, or lung cancers. The bone is the preferred site for metastases because of its highly vascular nature and extensive molecular signaling. A large number of bone tumor cases have been observed in an adolescent population experiencing a growth spurt and hormonal changes. Therefore, the treatment methodologies for bone tumors rarely involve the use of hormones as drugs but rather deal with hormone deprivation or inhibition. Though therapeutic approaches involving deprivation or replacement of hormones negatively affect bone health, the hormonal therapy alone or in combination with chemotherapeutic drugs offers a promising strategy for inhibition of bone tumors and improving the survival rates.

Acknowledgements

This article reflects collective intellectual wisdom of the authors. We thank Savitribai Phule Pune University, Pune, India, for providing the necessary infrastructure during the compilation of this chapter. We also thank our colleagues, whose work has been cited in this article, for their inspiration.

Conflict of interest

The authors declare no conflict of interest with relation to this study.

Author details

Geetanjali B. Tomar*, Jay R. Dave, Sayali S. Chandekar and Suhas T. Mhaske
Institute of Bioinformatics and Biotechnology, Savitribai Phule Pune University, Pune, India

*Address all correspondence to: geetanjalitomar13@gmail.com; joshigeet@gmail.com

References

[1] Dai X, Ma W, He X, Jha RK. Review of therapeutic strategies for osteosarcoma, chondrosarcoma, and Ewing's sarcoma. Medical Science Monitor. 2013;**17**:RA177-RA190. DOI: 10.12659/msm.881893

[2] Ibrahim T, Mercatali L, Amadori D. Bone and cancer: The osteoncology. Clinical Cases in Mineral and Bone Metabolism. 2013;**10**:121-123. DOI: 10.11138/ccmbm/2013.10.2.121

[3] Simmons JK, Hildreth BE, Supsavhad W, Elshafae SM, Hassan BB, Dirksen WP, et al. Animal models of bone metastasis. Veterinary Pathology. 2015;**52**:827-841. DOI: 10.1177/0300985815586223

[4] Gdowski AS, Ranjan A, Vishwanatha JK. Current concepts in bone metastasis, contemporary therapeutic strategies and ongoing clinical trials. Journal of Experimental & Clinical Cancer Research. 2017;**36**:1-13. DOI: 10.1186/s13046-017-0578-1

[5] Kakonen S-M, Mundy GR. Mechanisms of osteolytic bone metastases in breast carcinoma. Cancer. 2003;**97**:834-839. DOI: 10.1002/cncr.11132

[6] Nakai Y, Okamoto K, Terashima A, Ehata S, Nishida J, Imamura T, et al. Efficacy of an orally active small-molecule inhibitor of RANKL in bone metastasis. Bone Research. 2019;**7**:1-10. DOI: 10.1038/s41413-018-0036-5

[7] Schrage Y, Bovée J. Bone tumors: An overview. The Atlas of Genetics and Cytogenetics in Oncology and Haematology. 2011;**9**:166-170. DOI: 10.4267/2042/38197

[8] Chakarun CJ, Forrester DM, Gottsegen CJ, Patel DB, White EA, Matcuk GR. Giant cell tumor of bone: Review, mimics, and new developments in treatment. Radiographics. 2013;**33**: 197-211. DOI: 10.1148/rg.331125089

[9] Mak IWY, Turcotte RE, Ghert M. Parathyroid hormone-related protein (PTHrP) modulates adhesion, migration and invasion in bone tumor cells. Bone. 2013;**55**:198-207. DOI: 10.1016/j.bone.2013.02.020

[10] Evola FR, Costarella L, Pavone V, Caff G, Cannavò L, Sessa A, et al. Biomarkers of osteosarcoma, chondrosarcoma, and ewing sarcoma. Frontiers in Pharmacology. 2017;**8**:1-14

[11] Schwab JH, Springfield DS, Raskin KA, Mankin HJ, Hornicek FJ. What's new in primary bone tumors. Journal of Bone and Joint Surgery. 2012;**94**: 1913-1919. DOI: 10.2106/JBJS.L.00955

[12] Lindsey BA, Markel JE, Kleinerman ES. Osteosarcoma Overview. Rheumatology and Therapy. 2016;**4**:25-43. DOI: 10.1007/s40744-016-0050-2

[13] Li X, Yan ML, Yu Q. Identification of candidate drugs for the treatment of metastatic osteosarcoma through a subpathway analysis method. Oncology Letters. 2017;**13**:4378-4384. DOI: 10.3892/ol.2017.5953

[14] El-Naggar AM, Clarkson PW, Negri GL, Turgu B, Zhang F, Anglesio MS, et al. HACE1 is a potential tumor suppressor in osteosarcoma. Cell Death & Disease. 2019;**10**. DOI: 10.1038/s41419-018-1276-4

[15] Fang D, Yang H, Lin J, Teng Y, Jiang Y, Chen J, et al. 17β-Estradiol regulates cell proliferation, colony formation, migration, invasion and promotes apoptosis by upregulating miR-9 and thus degrades MALAT-1 in osteosarcoma cell MG-63 in an estrogen receptor-independent manner. Biochemical and Biophysical Research

Communications. 2015;**457**:500-506. DOI: 10.1016/j.bbrc.2014.12.114

[16] Yu PY, Gardner HL, Roberts R, Cam H, Hariharan S, Ren L, et al. Target specificity, in vivo pharmacokinetics, and efficacy of the putative STAT3 inhibitor LY5 in osteosarcoma, Ewing's sarcoma, and rhabdomyosarcoma. PLoS One. 2017;**12**:1-18. DOI: 10.1371/journal.pone.0181885

[17] Wu VM, Mickens J, Uskoković V. Bisphosphonate-functionalized hydroxyapatite nanoparticles for the delivery of the bromodomain inhibitor JQ1 in the treatment of osteosarcoma. ACS Applied Materials & Interfaces. 2017;**9**:25887-25904. DOI: 10.1021/acsami.7b08108

[18] Onimoe GI, Liu A, Lin L, Wei CC, Schwartz EB, Bhasin D, et al. Small molecules, LLL12 and FLLL32, inhibit STAT3 and exhibit potent growth suppressive activity in osteosarcoma cells and tumor growth in mice. Investigational New Drugs. 2012;**30**:916-926. DOI: 10.1007/s10637-011-9645-1

[19] Zhang S, Wang X, Gu Z, Wang L. Small molecule survivin inhibitor YM155 displays potent activity against human osteosarcoma cells. Cancer Investigation. 2016;**34**:401-407. DOI: 10.1080/07357907.2016.1212205

[20] Tovar C, Rosinski J, Filipovic Z, Higgins B, Kolinsky K, Hilton H, et al. Small-molecule MDM2 antagonists reveal aberrant p53 signaling in cancer: Implications for therapy. Proceedings of the National Academy of Sciences of the United States of America. 2006;**103**:1888-1893. DOI: 10.1073/pnas.0507493103

[21] Lillo Osuna MA, Garcia-Lopez J, El Ayachi I, Fatima I, Khalid AB, Kumpati J, et al. Activation of estrogen receptor alpha by decitabine inhibits osteosarcoma growth and metastasis. Cancer Research. 2018. DOI: 10.1158/0008-5472.can-18-1255

[22] Bone Cancer: Statistics [Internet]. Nov. 2018. Available from: https://www.cancer.net/cancer-types/bone-cancer/statistics

[23] Dorfman HD, Vanel D, Czerniak B, Park YK, Kotz R, Unni KK. WHO classification of tumours of bone: Introduction. World Health Organization. 2013:226-232

[24] Svoboda M, Hamilton G, Thalhammer T. Steroid hormone metabolizing enzymes in benign and malignant human bone tumors. Expert Opinion on Drug Metabolism & Toxicology. 2010;**6**:427-437. DOI: 10.1517/17425251003592129

[25] Guise TA. Molecular mechanisms of osteolytic bone metastases. Cancer. 1999;**88**:15-16. DOI: 10.1002/1097-0142(20000615)88:12+<2892::AID-CNCR2>3.0.CO;2-Y

[26] Nikitovic D, Kavasi RM, Berdiaki A, Papachristou DJ, Tsiaoussis J, Spandidos DA, et al. Parathyroid hormone/parathyroid hormone-related peptide regulate osteosarcoma cell functions: Focus on the extracellular matrix (review). Oncology Reports. 2016;**36**:1787-1792. DOI: 10.3892/or.2016.4986

[27] Weekes D, Kashima TG, Zandueta C, Perurena N, Thomas DP, Sunters A, et al. Regulation of osteosarcoma cell lung metastasis by the c-Fos/AP-1 target FGFR1. Oncogene. 2016;**35**:2852-2861. DOI: 10.1038/onc.2015.344

[28] Jiang M, Yan Y, Yang K, Liu Z, Qi J, Zhou H, et al. Small molecule nAS-E targeting cAMP response element binding protein (CREB) and CREB-binding protein interaction inhibits breast cancer bone metastasis. Journal of Cellular and Molecular Medicine. 2019;**23**:1224-1234. DOI: 10.1111/jcmm.14024

[29] Efstathiou E, Titus M, Wen S, Hoang A, Karlou M, Ashe R, et al. Molecular characterization of enzalutamide-treated bone metastatic castration-resistant prostate cancer. European Urology. 2015;**67**:53-60. DOI: 10.1016/j.eururo.2014.05.005

[30] D'Oronzo S, Brown J, Coleman R. The value of biomarkers in bone metastasis. European Journal of Cancer Care. 2017;**26**:1-10. DOI: 10.1111/ecc.12725

[31] Chirgwin JM, Wong DH, Corey E, Higgins LS, Stebbins EG, Guise TA, et al. Basic mechanisms responsible for osteolytic and osteoblastic bone metastases. Clinical Cancer Research. 2006;**12**:6213s-6216s. DOI: 10.1158/1078-0432.ccr-06-1007

[32] Bado I, Gugala Z, Fuqua SAW, Zhang XH-F. Estrogen receptors in breast and bone: From virtue of remodeling to vileness of metastasis. Oncogene. 2017;**36**:4527-4537. DOI: 10.1038/onc.2017.94

[33] Bone Cancer: Introduction [Internet]. 2018. Available from: https://www.cancer.net/cancer-types/bone-cancer/introduction

[34] Logothetis CJ, Lin SH. Osteoblasts in prostate cancer metastasis to bone. Nature Reviews. Cancer. 2005;**5**:21-28. DOI: 10.1038/nrc1528

[35] Kushlinskii NE, Timofeev YS, Solov'ev YN, Gerstein ES, Lyubimova NV, Bulycheva IV. Components of the RANK/RANKL/OPG system, IL-6, IL-8, IL-16, MMP-2, and calcitonin in the sera of patients with bone tumors. Bulletin of Experimental Biology and Medicine. 2014;**157**:520-523. DOI: 10.1007/s10517-014-2605-y

[36] Suva LJ, Washam C, Nicholas RW, Griffin RJ. Bone metastasis: Mechanisms and therapeutic opportunities. Nature Reviews Endocrinology. 2011;7:208-218. DOI: 10.1038/nrendo.2010.227

[37] Duan Z, Zhang J, Ye S, Shen J, Choy E, Cote G, et al. A-770041 reverses paclitaxel and doxorubicin resistance in osteosarcoma cells. BMC Cancer. 2014;**14**:1-11. DOI: 10.1186/1471-2407-14-681

[38] Macedo F, Ladeira K, Pinho F, Saraiva N, Bonito N, Pinto L, et al. Bone metastases: An overview. Oncology Reviews. 2017;**11**:43-49. DOI: 10.4081/oncol.2017.321

[39] Mantalaris A, Panoskaltsis N, Sakai Y, Bourne P, Chang C, Messing EM, et al. Localization of androgen receptor expression in human bone marrow. The Journal of Pathology. 2001;**193**:361-366. DOI: 10.1002/1096-9896(0000)9999:9999<::AID-PATH803>3.0.CO;2-W

[40] Ito Y, Sadar MD. Enzalutamide and blocking androgen receptor in advanced prostate cancer: Lessons learnt from the history of drug development of antiandrogens. Research and Reports in Urology. 2018;**10**:23-32. DOI: 10.2147/RRU.S157116

[41] Deivaraju C, Temple HT, Block N, Robinson P, Schally AV. LHRH receptor expression in sarcomas of bone and soft tissue. Hormone Molecular Biology and Clinical Investigation. 2016;**28**:105-111. DOI: 10.1515/hmbci-2016-0001

[42] Langley RE, Kynaston HG, Alhasso AA, Duong T, Paez EM, Jovic G, et al. A randomised comparison evaluating changes in bone mineral density in advanced prostate cancer: Luteinising hormone-releasing hormone agonists versus transdermal oestradiol. European Urology: European Association of Urology. 2016;**69**:1016-1025. DOI: 10.1016/j.eururo.2015.11.030

[43] Diaz-Convalia E, Arrabal-Polo MA. Cano-Garcia M del C, Dominguez-Amillo A, Canales-Casco N, Arrabal-Martin M. Risk of renal stone formation in patients treated with luteinising hormone-releasing hormone analogues for prostate

cancer: Importance of bone metabolism and urine calcium. International Urology and Nephrology. 2018;**50**:419-425. DOI: 10.1007/s11255-018-1793-1

[44] de Bono JS, Logothetis CJ, Molina A, Fizazi K, North S, Chu L, et al. Abiraterone and increased survival in metastatic prostate cancer. The New England Journal of Medicine. 2011;**364**:1995-2005. DOI: 10.1056/NEJMoa1014618

[45] Gravanis I, Lopez AS, Hemmings RJ, Jimenez JC, Garcia-Carbonero R, Gallego IG, et al. The European medicines agency review of abiraterone for the treatment of metastatic castration-resistant prostate cancer in adult men after docetaxel chemotherapy and in chemotherapy-naive disease: Summary of the scientific assessment of the committee for medicinal products for human use. The Oncologist. 2013;**18**:1032-1042. DOI: 10.1634/theoncologist.2013-0092

[46] Body J-J, Casimiro S, Costa L. Targeting bone metastases in prostate cancer: improving clinical outcome. Nature Reviews Urology. 2015;**12**: 340-356. DOI: 10.1038/nrurol.2015.90

[47] El-Amm J, Patel N, Freeman A, Aragon-Ching JB. Metastatic castration-resistant prostate cancer: Critical review of enzalutamide. Clinical Medicine Insights: Oncology. 2013;**7**:235-245. DOI: 10.4137/CMO.S11670

[48] Miki K, Sasaki H, Kido M, Takahashi H, Aoki M, Egawa S. A comparative study on the efficacies of gonadotropin-releasing hormone (GnRH) agonist and GnRH antagonist in neoadjuvant androgen deprivation therapy combined with transperineal prostate brachytherapy for localized prostate cancer. BMC Cancer. 2016;**16**: 1-7. DOI: 10.1186/s12885-016-2737-8

[49] Kashiwabara T, Suda S. Usefulness of combined androgen blockade therapy with gonadotropin-releasing hormone antagonist for bone metastatic prostate cancer with pretreatment prostate-specific antigen level ≥ 50 ng/mL. BMC Cancer. 2018;**18**:1-11. DOI: 10.1186/s12885-018-4541-0

[50] Yu EY, Getzenberg RH, Coss CC, Gittelman MM, Keane T, Tutrone R, et al. Selective estrogen receptor alpha agonist GTx-758 decreases testosterone with reduced side effects of androgen deprivation therapy in men with advanced prostate cancer. European Urology: European Association of Urology. 2015;**67**:334-341. DOI: 10.1016/j.eururo.2014.06.011

[51] Hofbauer LC, Rachner TD, Coleman RE, Jakob F. Endocrine aspects of bone metastases. The Lancet Diabetes and Endocrinology. 2014;**2**:500-512. DOI: 10.1016/S2213-8587(13)70203-1

[52] He S, Nelson ER. 27-Hydroxycholesterol, an endogenous selective estrogen receptor modulator. Maturitas. 2017;**104**:29-35. DOI: 10.1016/j.maturitas.2017.07.014

[53] Salvatori L, Caporuscio F, Coroniti G, Starace G, Frati L, Russo MA, et al. Down-regulation of epidermal growth factor receptor induced by estrogens and phytoestrogens promotes the differentiation of U2OS human osteosarcoma cells. Journal of Cellular Physiology. 2009;**220**:35-44. DOI: 10.1002/jcp.21724

[54] Chrzan BG, Bradford PG. Phytoestrogens activate estrogen receptor β1 and estrogenic responses in human breast and bone cancer cell lines. Molecular Nutrition & Food Research. 2007;**51**:171-177. DOI: 10.1002/mnfr.200600091

[55] Rajah TT, Peine KJ, Du N, Serret CA, Drews NR. Physiological concentrations of genistein and 17β-estradiol inhibit MDA-MB-231 breast cancer cell growth by increasing

BAX/BCL-2 and reducing pERK1/2. Anticancer Research. 2012;**32**:1181-1191

[56] Wang W, Belosay A, Yang X, Hartman JA, Song H, Iwaniec UT, et al. Effects of letrozole on breast cancer micro-metastatic tumor growth in bone and lung in mice inoculated with murine 4T1 cells. Clinical & Experimental Metastasis. 2016;**33**:475-485. DOI: 10.1007/s10585-016-9792-z

[57] Ariazi EA, Leitao A, Oprea TI, Chen B, Louis T, Bertucci AM, et al. Exemestane's 17-hydroxylated metabolite exerts biological effects as an androgen. Molecular Cancer Therapeutics. 2007;**6**:2817-2827. DOI: 10.1158/1535-7163.mct-07-0312

[58] Bartels S, Christgen M, Luft A, Persing S, Jödecke K, Lehmann U, et al. Estrogen receptor (ESR1) mutation in bone metastases from breast cancer. Modern Pathology. 2018;**31**:56-61. DOI: 10.1038/modpathol.2017.95

[59] Kang E, Cho JH, Choi J-H, Yoo H-W. Etiology and therapeutic outcomes of children with gonadotropin-independent precocious puberty. Annals of Pediatric Endocrinology & Metabolism. 2016;**21**:136. DOI: 10.6065/apem.2016.21.3.136

[60] Gorska M, Wyszkowska RM, Kuban-Jankowska A, Wozniak M. Impact of apparent antagonism of estrogen receptor β by fulvestrant on anticancer activity of 2-methoxyestradiol. Anticancer Research [Internet]. 2016;**36**:2217-2226. Available from: http://www.ncbi.nlm.nih.gov/pubmed/27127126

[61] Holen I, Walker M, Nutter F, Fowles A, Evans CA, Eaton CL, et al. Oestrogen receptor positive breast cancer metastasis to bone: inhibition by targeting the bone microenvironment in vivo. Clinical & Experimental Metastasis. 2016;**33**:211-224. DOI: 10.1007/s10585-015-9770-x

[62] Zhou Q, Shen L, Liu C, Liu C, Chen H, Liu J. The effects of estradiol and glucocorticoid on human osteosarcoma cells: Similarities and differences. Anticancer Research. 2016;**36**:1683-1691

Chapter 3

Role of Pineal Hormone Melatonin in a Woman's Life: From Conception to Decline of Life

Elena N. Usoltseva and Marina V. Danilova

Abstract

In the presented article, we cover the issues concerning physiology of secretion of pineal hormone melatonin and its role in the vital processes of a body. Focus is given to melatonin effect on the female reproductive system, its participation in the aging process, and formation of pathological menopause. The article also presents research data on the effectiveness of the melatonin drug when tackling climacteric syndrome. It is revealed that according to the available literature up to date there is no information about the standards of secretion of melatonin for women of different age groups, and the lack of secretion of melatonin can be judged by clinical manifestations and also when compared with groups of healthy women. The issues of the melatonin drug application at various complications of pregnancy and gynecological diseases remain unclear. Long-term intake of melatonin to treat pathologic menopause is still to be discussed.

Keywords: women, pineal gland, melatonin, 6-sulfatoxymelatonin

1. Introduction

Melatonin is a principal hormone produced by pineal cells in the pineal gland located in the cerebrum center behind the third ventricle (**Figure 1**). This endocrine gland consists of two cell types: pineal cells (which dominate and produce indolamines, mainly represented by melatonin, and peptides, such as arginine vasotocin) and neuroglia cells. The information received from neurons and modified by means

Key points

1. Melatonin functions in the human body are very diverse, and its normal secretion is extremely important for the preservation of somatic health.

2. The important role of melatonin in the formation of the reproductive function of women, the formation of a two-phase cycle, high-quality ovulation and fertilization, prevention of violations of a number of gynecological and obstetric pathologies.

Currently there are convincing data on the role of melatonin in the onset of menopause, the formation of climacteric syndrome, depression, osteoporosis, dyslipidemia, menopausal metabolic syndrome and cardiovascular diseases, and breast cancer in women in perimenopausal and postmenopausal women.

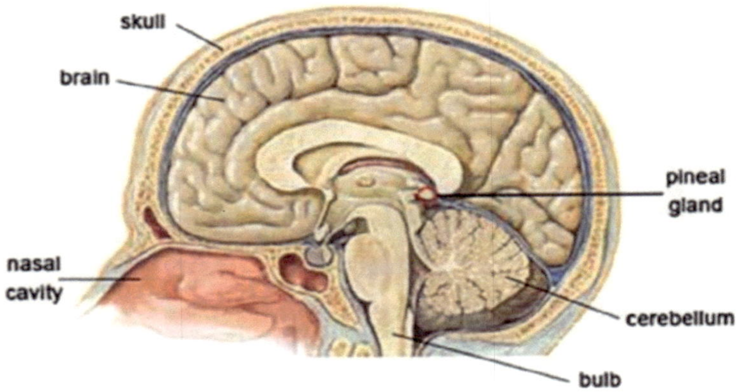

Figure 1.
Anatomical location for pineal body.

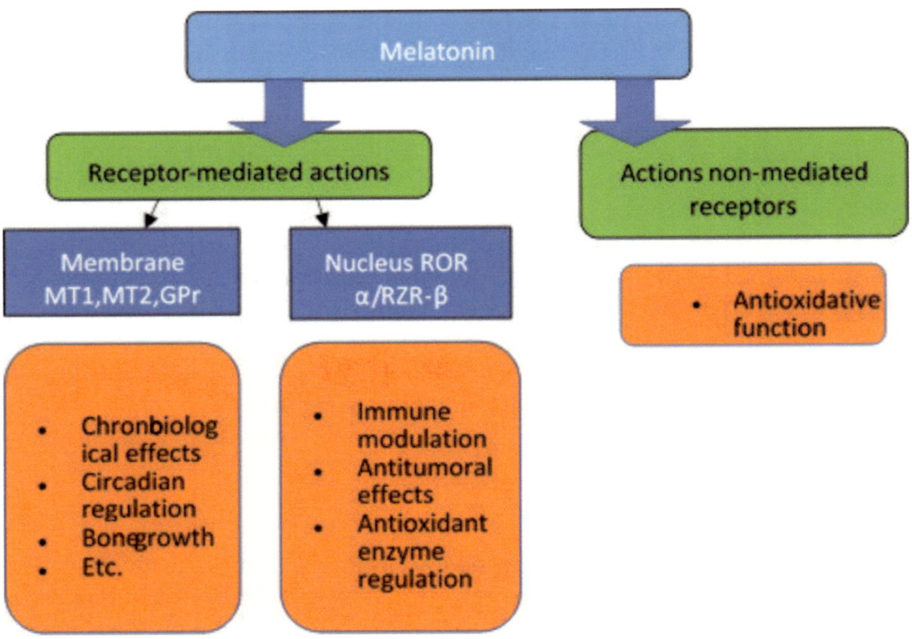

Figure 2.
Melatonin mechanisms of action.

of night and daylight intensity transforms in the pineal gland into chemical signals. Receiving the information about luminosity the pineal gland turns it into endocrine response by producing melatonin, which is a biogenic amine pertaining to the indole class, based on its chemical structure. Melatonin is a derivant of biogenic amine serotonin, which in its turn is synthesized from the amino acid tryptophan, received with food. Activity of ferments participating in serotonin transformation into melatonin is suppressed by lighting—that is why this hormone can be produced only during hours of darkness [1].

Melatonin is mainly released to the cerebrospinal fluid (liquor), getting from there to the blood flow and afterwards easily allocating itself in various organs and tissues due to good lipophilic properties [2]. Key effects of melatonin are connected with the action on membrane receptors—*MT*1 and *MT*2. They relate to a group of receptors connected with G-protein. These receptors are responsible for chronobiological effects and regulation of circadian rhythm and are widely distributed in different organs and tissues. Melatonin receptor presentation in the reproductive organs and receptors to sexual hormones in the epiphysis enables drawing the conclusion that melatonin plays an important role in regulation of reproductive aspect (**Figure 2**).

In the same way, the nuclear receptors of melatonin *ROR*-α/*RZR*-β have been discovered. It is evident that many immune-stimulating and antitumoral effects are mediated by them.

Antioxidative function of melatonin is based on the receptor action, but this hormone is able to directly withdraw free radicals without receptor actuation [3].

Russian scientists discovered that apart from epiphyseal melatonin, there is an extrapineal one that is formed in different gastrointestinal tracts and other organs: liver, kidneys, supramental capsules, gall bladder, ovaries, endometrium, placenta, thymus, white blood cells, thrombocytes, and endothelium. Biologic action of the extrapineal melatonin is carried out right where it is synthesized [1].

2. Melatonin main physiological functions and its role in maintaining human health

During the recent years, new data on the mechanisms providing for the integral interaction among the nervous, immune, and endocrine systems have been received. Presumably, pineal gland is an integrator of such interaction, while its main hormone, melatonin, takes part in regulation of the activity of central and vegetative nervous systems, endocrine organs, and immune system. The performed investigations have demonstrated that melatonin fulfills an extremely wide range of physiological functions: biorhythmic and immunomodulatory processes, thermal control and sleep onset, and antioxidative and anti-stress effects [3]. Hormone secretion starts on the third month of infant development and reaches its peak during the first years (not later than at the age of 5). Before puberty, melatonin synthesis remains at a constantly high level [4]. During the age of 11–14, due to the fact that the pineal gland reduces melatonin production, the hormone mechanisms of sexual development are launched. The next significant reduction in activity occurs simultaneously with menopause onset—at the age of 45–60. With the aging progression, along with decrease in basal level, melatonin secretion peaks are getting lower [1]. During daytime melatonin concentration in the blood serum remains low (10–20 pg/ml), while during the night hours it grows considerably (80,120 pg/ml) and reaches its maximum value between midnight and 3–5 a.m. Melatonin secretion usually starts at 9 p.m. and terminates at 7–9 a.m. Melatonin metabolites are found in urine: 6-sulfatoxymelatonin (80–90%) and 6-hydroxyglucuronide (10–20%) corresponding to the circadian rhythm that is very close to the rhythm of melatonin secretion [5].

A new science, biorhythmology, introduced the notion of desynchronosis—clinically very important—that means ill-being or pathological syndrome, which is connected with the unbalance of circadian rhythms. A degree of desynchronosis is defined by the quantity and rhythm of melatonin production during the day and night. It has been determined that when a somatic disease goes hard or aggravates, melatonin production is getting worse, and its night indicator is getting closer to the day value [6]. Disturbed melatonin secretion finds its clinical manifestation in tiredness, indisposition, sleep disorder, and sometimes aggravation of a chronic disease or even appearance of a new one. Desynchronosis condition is exemplified by jet lag syndrome caused by rapid long-distance transmeridian travel [7].

It is generally known that melatonin has an antidepressant function. However, foreign colleagues stated disturbed circadian rhythm of melatonin secretion experienced by patients with depression during a menopause along with its increase during the morning hours as compared with women in good health that also has impact on sleep, level of follicle-stimulating hormone, and body mass index [8]. A connection was established between sleep disorder and melatonin reduction in female saliva during perimenopause without registering such pattern among women in postmenopause [9].

Therefore, melatonin functions in a human body are quite diversified, and its normal secretion is highly important for maintaining human health in a contemporary world.

3. Melatonin involvement into hormonal regulation of female reproductive system functions and its aging

In 1963 R.J. Wurtman et al. reported for the first time that exogenic intake of melatonin causes weight reduction in female rat ovaries. Since those times many evidences that pineal gland and its main hormone, melatonin, influence reproductive function have been received. Studies showed that neurons in preoptic and mediobasal areas of hypothalamus and hypophysis represented the main points, through which melatonin produced its reproductive action. The main physiological effect of melatonin lies in the slowdown of gonadotrophin secretion, with greater suppression of the lutenizing hormone (LH) by melatonin rather than the follicle-stimulating one. Negative correlation is registered between melatonin level at night and lutenizing hormone concentration. In addition, secretion of other tropic hormones of hypophysis anterior lobe (such as corticotrophin, thyrotropin, somatotropin) is reduced, though to a lesser extent. Melatonin can be called a universal inhibitor of endocrine function in a female body [10].

Melatonin takes part in regulation of many vital physiological processes, such as puberty and genital formation, menstrual cycle, and aging of reproductive system. High level of nocturnal melatonin was found in children with delayed puberty, while among children having accelerated puberty, a decrease in melatonin secretion at night was noted. High levels of melatonin among children produce a dominating effect on pulsatile gonadotropin secretion, ovary function, and puberty [4].

Abnormal levels of melatonin in blood are connected with a number of malfunctions in the system "hypothalamus—hypophysis—ovaries." This gives boost to precocious puberty or its delay and formation of hypothalamic or hypergonadotropic amenorrhea. Therefore, melatonin may have indirect influence on the function of reproductive glands through its intervention into the secretion of gonadotropin-releasing hormone and/or secretion of gonadotrophins. Some data demonstrate that melatonin can also be synthesized in reproductive glands. Decreased melatonin secretion in summer coincides with higher fertility among women living in the Northern Hemisphere [11].

Based on these data, it was presupposed that melatonin could be a part of events preceding activation of hypothalamus-ovary axis during a puberty period [12]. Non-serial MRI of female head region helped register a reliable decrease in pineal gland volume during the ovulatory phase as well as while perimenopause. It indicates pineal gland involvement into "turning off" female reproductive function [13].

Melatonin may also produce direct influence on ovaries. High level of melatonin was found in preovulatory follicular fluid with triple concentration as compared to blood. Connecting areas of iodine melatonin were identified in human cells of granulosis and preovulatory follicles.

Antioxidative effect of melatonin is considered to be the most prominent one. It has been determined that melatonin ties free radicals of oxygen and at the same time stimulates enzymatic systems and SOD and possesses protective properties in relation to free-radical damage of DNA [14].

It's generally known that macrofags, neutrophils, and vascular endothelium cells located in follicles produce AOS during ovulation. Despite the fact that AOS (active oxygen species) participate in breaking follicles, potentially they may damage an ovum and granulosis lutein cells. AOS inhibit progesterone production by lutein cells due to inhibition of steroidogenesis enzymes and transport intracellular protein. Melatonin is an important antioxidant in ovary follicles and enables progesterone synthesis by luteal cells [15]. Research outcomes have shown that melatonin intake leads to increased concentration of this hormone in follicular fluid and reduced oxidative damage inside follicles, thus raising a chance of fertilization and pregnancy [16, 17]. Melatonin intake also improved progesterone synthesis among women with infertility issues caused by insufficiency of the cycle luteal phase [18].

Pregnancy and acts of delivery are characterized by deep alterations in the endocrine profile of a female body as well as in pineal gland operation. In the case of physiological pregnancy, increased melatonin excretion with urine is marked, while just before an act of delivery its level plummets.

Decreased melatonin level is noted in the case of threatening miscarriage [4].

At the same time, many scientists speak about the great importance of melatonin in the body aging process. It is also pointed out that from the age of 45, melatonin starts to decline steadily till the end of human life. Numerous studies have demonstrated the correlation between melatonin synthesis and menopause onset [19]. The second decrease in melatonin level may be related to involutory processes in pineal gland [13].

In a placebo-controlled clinical study, it was established that there was a connection between decreased content of nocturnal melatonin in saliva and menopause onset, while intake of 3 mg of melatonin by female patients during perimenopause on a daily basis for 6 months eliminates hormonal and neurovegetative disorders and recovers menstruation cycle and thyroid function [20].

Women in postmenopause had lower concentration of melatonin in blood serum as compared to women in perimenopause, with a shorter duration of melatonin secretion in postmenopause as a rule, while melatonin synthesis peak time (acrophase) was almost the same. A pattern was determined that as melatonin secretion peak occurs later among women in perimenopause, anxiety level gets higher ($p = 0.022$), and as melatonin secretion continues for a longer period, the quality of life among patients gets better ($p < 0.001$) [21].

Some scientists suggest using melatonin drugs at the first stage of climacteric disorder treatment even before the start of hormonal therapy of menopause [4]. Moreover, in a double-blind placebo-controlled clinical study, it was determined that prescription of menopause hormonal therapy to postmenopausal women shifts melatonin secretion peak time without changing the melatonin level in the blood serum, which requires further research [21]. Other authors did not found in their research analyses devoted to alternative therapy for climacteric disorders any convincing data on hot flash arresting by melatonin drug [22].

4. Melatonin lipid metabolism

A growing number of evidences are emerging, which point to melatonin involvement into lipid metabolism. The study of H. Tamura was devoted to melatonin influence on lipid metabolism among women in perimenopause and postmenopause. A negative correlation was established between nocturnal melatonin and total cholesterol level, low-density lipoprotein, and positive correlation with high-density lipoprotein. No correlation was found between nocturnal melatonin and triglyceride level in blood. These findings show that melatonin drug prescription may represent a new approach to the correction of lipid metabolism and prevention of cardiovascular diseases during perimenopause and postmenopause [23]. Other scientists determined that melatonin improves lipid profile (leads to a reduced level of low-density lipoprotein) and fulfills antioxidant protection [24].

Under a study led by L.I. Maltseva [25], scientists analyzed melatonin role in the development of climacteric syndrome and its effectiveness for treating pathological climacterium. Russian scientists established that the level of 6-sulfatoxymelatonin in a 24-h urine among patients with severe climacteric syndrome amounts to 35.09 ± 3.5 ng/ml, medium severity (44.01 ± 7.92 ng/ml), and mild climacteric syndrome (45.91 ± 12.42 ng/ml) (1.7 times lower as compared to women in good health). Accordingly, secretory function of hypophysis is altered in various ways. Women with low level of 6-sulfatoxymelatonin in a 24-h urine show significant growth of both gonadotropic hormones—follicle-stimulating and luteinizing hormones—in a proportional way. A research showed that women had a high level of catecholamines (adrenaline and noradrenaline) with its degree being dependent on climacteric syndrome severity. It was also determined that women in perimenopausal age have increased the level of atherogenic fractions of blood lipids on the background of lower melatonin level.

Scientists came to the conclusion that melatonin acts as a modifier of alterations which occur with the development of climacteric disorders and influence hormonal, mediating, and biochemical indicators of the female body. Women with mild climacteric syndrome taking 3 mg of melatonin per day as monotherapy demonstrated during the repeated evaluation of clinical, hormonal, and biochemical indicators after 1 month a positive dynamics of all indicators. The blood hormone level was close to reference values, follicle-stimulating hormone level dropped by 2.29 times, luteinizing hormone level by 2.1 times. Values of melatonin sulfate in a 24-h urine grew by 2.64 times and were close as never to the reference values 27.95 ± 7.92...73.95 ± 24.85 ng/ml. However more significant alterations were noted for the severe climacteric syndrome without any side effects when melatonin treatment and menopause hormonal therapy were used together [25].

5. Menopause and sleep disturbance

Japanese scientists stated that estradiol level was firmly higher among women that worked night shifts and went to sleep later than 1 a.m. as compared to women that slept at night, with the level of serum testosterone and DHEA-sulfate unaffected, while 6-sulfatoxymelatonin concentration in urine was lower among the first group patients. Similar hormonal disruptions among postmenopausal women experiencing sleep disorder represent serious risk factors of breast cancer [26]. Singapore Chinese Health Study (2008) also showed that among women in postmenopause, the risk of breast cancer gets lower when sleep duration increases (p = 0.047). When sleep duration exceeds 9 h, a relative risk equals to 0.67 (95% confidence interval 0.4–1.1) as compared to women with a sleep duration of 6 h or less. At that, melatonin level was higher by 42% when sleep duration was 9 h or more. Such pattern was registered for women with normal weight (body mass index of 23.2 kg/m), p = 0.024 [27]. American scientists proved through a largescale prospective analysis that among women with 6-sulfatoxymelatonin content within the upper quartile, there were fewer with invasive breast cancer than among those whose values were within the bottom quartile [28]. It was established that the increased concentration of 6-sulfatoxymelatonin in the morning urine portion was statistically related to a lower risk of breast cancer (ratio of chances for upper and lower quartiles of 6-sulfatoxymelatonin level 0.62; 95% confidence interval 0.41–0.95; $p = 0.004$) [29].

C.G. Harrod and his colleagues made an assumption that a growing risk of cerebrovascular disease registered among menopausal women can be to some extent explained by changes in the level of circulating melatonin and estrogens and their modulating influence on biologic activity of endothelial cells, including vascular tone regulation, leukocytes adhesion, and angiogenesis. This hypothesis is confirmed by numerous studies demonstrating the braking effect of melatonin and estrogens on vessel tone, neuroprotection, and expression of receptors [30].

Increased melatonin secretion in the morning is more typical for menopausal patients with depression than women in good health. Moreover, menopause duration, level of the follicle-stimulating hormone, sleep end time, and body mass index may lead to alterations in melatonin secretion when suffering from depression during a menopause [8].

6. Melatonin effects on bone metabolism

At present a relation between melatonin and skeleton is known. Melatonin may produce an effect on bone tissue which manifests itself in bone tissue formation with osteoblasts and/or hindering bone resorption with osteoclasts. The study of K. Satomura et al. [31] confirms the melatonin (*Mel1*) receptor expression in human osteoblasts and tendency of its level reduction with aging. It is also demonstrated that melatonin can have a boosting effect on proliferation and differentiation of human osteoblasts [32]. Through a controlled randomized trial (2012), exogenous melatonin effect on bone tissue density was revealed. Bone tissue condition was controlled in two ways—bone tissue density estimation and bone marker determination. There was no considerable improvement noted in terms of bone tissue density in T points or as compared with placebo. An average change in the activity of bone resorption marker, N-telopeptide (NTX), in this study did not differ much inside and between the groups. Similarly, the average change in the activity of bone formation marker, osteocalcin, did not show any remarkable differences either inside a group or between groups. However, NTX to osteocalcin ratio followed a downward trend among the women who took melatonin as compared to placebo. It is quite important because among menopausal women, this ratio is known to increase so that osteoclasts activity outstrips osteoblast activity, which leads to a loss of bone mass. Probably, decreased level of nocturnal melatonin that occurs during a menopause causes hormonal unbalance and perimenopause symptoms, including the loss in bone mass. These data prove that melatonin intake may enable the balancing of bone resorption and formation processes, potentially preventing fast loss of bone mass attributed to a menopausal period [33].

Melatonin inhibits resorption activity by reducing RANKL-mediated osteoclastogenesis and therefore decreases bone resorption. Melatonin also protects from losing bone mass induced by free radicals, which occurs in the case of extreme bone resorption, due to its powerful antioxidative properties [34, 35]. In addition to its direct effect on the bone tissue, melatonin can produce an indirect influence on bone metabolism through the hypothalamus-pituitary axis, by suppressing levels of follicle-stimulating hormone and estrogen and increasing the level of progesterone. In contrast to the follicle-stimulating hormone, melatonin has positive correlation with progesterone level. Progesterone is known to influence on the mineral density of bone tissue, especially on osteoblast differentiation [36]. Reduced level of progesterone during a perimenopause may lead to the decreasing of bone tissue density because of osteoblasts loss.

7. Conclusion

Therefore, melatonin role in a female body is quite significant from the moment of birth till the last breath. It is revealed that up to the present time according to the literature data there is no information about the standards of secretion of melatonin for women of different age groups, and the lack of secretion of melatonin can be judged by clinical manifestations, and also when compared with groups of healthy women. The issues of using melatonin treatment for different cases of pregnancy complications and gynecological disorders remain unclear. Long-term intake of melatonin to treat pathological menopause is still to be discussed.

Author details

Elena N. Usoltseva[1] and Marina V. Danilova[2*]

1 Department of Obstetrics and Gynecology, South Ural State Medical University, Health Ministry of Russian Federation, Chelyabinsk, Russia

2 City Clinical Hospital № 1, Chelyabinsk, Russia

*Address all correspondence to: danilova-mv@bk.ru

References

[1] Anisimov VN. Melatonin—Its Role in a Human Body, Clinical Application. SPb.: Sistema; 2007

[2] Arushanyan EB. Pregnancy and pineal gland. Ros Vestn, akush-gin. 2012;**6**:29-34

[3] Bespyatykh AY, Brodskiy VY, Burlakova OV, et al. In: Repport SI, Golichenkov VA, editors. Melatonin: Theory and practice. M.: Medpraktika-M; 2009

[4] Anisimov VN, Vinogradova IA. Aging of Female Reproductive System and Melatonin. SPb., Sistema; 2008

[5] Karasek M, Winczyk K. Melatonin in human. Journal of Physiology and Pharmacology. 2006;**57**(5):19-39

[6] Ragosin ON, Bochkarev MV. Effect of the Northern Region Modified Photoperiodism on Normal and Abnormal Human Biological Rhythms: Guide on Chronobiology and Chronomedicine. M: MIA; 2012. pp. 119-136

[7] Vosko AM, Colwell CS, Avidan AY. Jet lag syndrome: Circadian organization, pathophysiology, and management strategies. Nature and Science of Sleep. 2010;**2**: 187-198

[8] Parry BL, Meliska CJ, Sorenson DL, et al. Increased melatonin and delayed offset in menopausal depression: Role of years past menopause, folliclestimulating hormone, sleep end time, and body mass index. Journal of Clinical Endocrinology and Metabolism. 2008;**93**(1):54-60

[9] Kolesnikova LI, Madaeva IM, Semenova NV, et al. Pathogenic role of melatonin in sleep disorders in menopausal women. Bulletin of Experimental Biology and Medicine. 2013;**156**(1):104-106

[10] Brzezinski A, Lynch HJ, Wurtman RJ, Seibel MM. Possible contribution of melatonin to the timing of the luteinizing hormone surge. New England Journal of Medicine. 1987;**316**:1550-1551

[11] Boczek-Leszczyk E, Juszczak M. The influence of melatonin on human reproduction. Polski Merkuriusz Lekarski. 2007;**23**(134):128-130

[12] Brzezinski A. Melatonin and human reproduction: Why the effect is so elusive? In: Pandi-Perumal SR, Cardinali DP, editors. Molecules to Therapy. New York: Nova Science Publishers; 2007. pp. 219-225

[13] Ivanov SV. Menopause is a key aspect of aging: Role of pineal gland. Advances in Gerontology. 2007;**4**(20):19-24

[14] Hardeland R. Antioxidative protection by melatonin: Multiplicity of mechanisms from radical detoxification to radical avoidance. Endocrine. 2005;**27**(2):119-130

[15] Tamura H, Takasaki A, Taketani T, et al. Melatonin and female reproduction. Journal of Obstetrics and Gynaecology Research. 2014;**40**(1):1-11

[16] Tamura H, Nakamura Y, Korkmaz A, et al. Melatonin and the ovary: Physiological and pathophysiological implications. Fertility and Sterility. 2009;**92**:328-343

[17] Tamura H, Takasaki A, Miwa I, et al. Oxidative stress impairs oocyte quality and melatonin protects oocytes from free radical damage and improves fertilization rate. Journal of Pineal Research. 2008;**44**:280-287

[18] Taketani T, Tamura H, Takasaki A, et al. Protective role of melatonin in progesterone production by human

luteal cells. Journal of Pineal Research. 2011;**51**:207-213

[19] Diaz BL, Llaneza PC. Endocrine regulation of the course of menopause by oral melatonin: First case report. Menopause. 2008;**15**:388-392

[20] Bellipanni G, Di Marzo F, Blasi F, Di Marzo A. Effects of melatonin in perimenopausal and menopausal women: Our personal experience. Annals of the New York Academy of Sciences. 2005;**1057**:393-402

[21] Toffol E, Kalleinen N, Haukka J, et al. Melatonin in peri-menopausal and postmenopausal women: Associations with mood, sleep, climacteric symptoms, and quality of life. Menopause. 2014;**21**(5):493-500

[22] Kelley KW, Carroll DG. Evaluating the evidence for over-the-counter alternatives for relief of hot flashes in menopausal women. Journal of the American Pharmacists Association. 2010;**50**(5):106-115

[23] Tamura H, Nakamura Y, Narimatsu A, et al. Melatonin treatment in peri- and postmenopausal women elevates serum high-density lipoprotein cholesterol levels without influencing total cholesterol levels. Journal of Pineal Research. 2008;**45**:101-105

[24] Kozirog M, Poliwczak AR, Duchnowicz P, et al. Melatonin treatment improves blood pressure, lipid profile, and parameters of oxidative stress in patients with metabolic syndrome. Journal of Pineal Research. 2011;**50**:261-266

[25] Maltseva LI, Gafarova EA, Garipova GH. Melatonin role in reproductive glands function regulation and possibility of its use for pathological climacteric symptoms treatment. Advances in Gerontology. 2007;**4**(20):68-74

[26] Nagata C, Nagao Y, Yamamoto S, et al. Light exposure at night, urinary 6sulfatoxymelatonin, and serum estrogens and androgens in postmenopausal Japanese women. Cancer Epidemiology, Biomarkers & Prevention. 2008;**17**(6):1418-1423

[27] Wu AH, Wang R, Koh WP. et al, Sleep duration, melatonin and breast cancer among Chinese women in Singapore. Carcinogenesis. 2008;**29**(6):1244-1248

[28] Schernhammer ES, Berrino F, Krogh V, et al. Urinary 6-sulfatoxymelatonin levels and risk of breast cancer in post-menopausal women. Journal of the National Cancer Institute. 2008;**100**(12):898-905

[29] Schernhammer ES, Hankinson SE. Urinary melatonin levels and postmenopausal breast cancer risk in the nurses' health study cohort. Cancer Epidemiology, Biomarkers & Prevention. 2009;**18**(1):74-79

[30] Harrod CG, Bendok BR, Hunt Batjer H. Interactions between mela tonin and estrogen may regulate cerebrovascular function in women: Clinical implications for the effective use of HRT during menopause and aging. Medical Hypotheses. 2008;**70**(1):213

[31] Satomura K, Tobiume S, Tokuyama R, Yamasaki Y, et al. Melatonin at pharmacological doses enhances human osteoblastic differentiation in vitro and promotes mouse cortical bone formation in vivo. Journal of Pineal Research. 2007 Apr;**42**(3):231-239

[32] Park KH, Kang JW, Lee EM, et al. Melatonin promotes osteoblastic differentiation through the BMP/ERK/Wnt signaling pathways. Journal of Pineal Research. 2011;**51**:187-194

[33] Kotlarczyk MP, Lassila HC, O'Neil CK, et al. Melatonin osteoporosis

prevention study (MOPS): A randomized, double-blind, placebo-controlled study examining the effects of melatonin on bone health and quality of life in perimenopausal women. Journal of Pineal Research. 2012;**52**(4):414-426

[34] Galano A, Tan DX, Reiter RJ. Melatonin as a natural ally against oxidative stress: A physicochemical examination. Journal of Pineal Research. 2011;**51**:1-16

[35] Sanchez-Barcelo EJ, Mediavilla MD, Tan DX, et al. Scientific basis for the potential use of melatonin in bone diseases: Osteoporosis and adolescent idiopathic scoliosis. Journal of Osteoporosis. 1 Jun 2010;**2010**:830231. DOI: 10.4061/2010/830231

[36] Seifert-Klauss V, Prior JC. Progesterone and bone: Actions promoting bone health in women. Journal of Osteoporosis. 31 Oct 2010;**2010**:845180. DOI: 10.4061/2010/845180

Chapter 4

Symptoms of Menopause

Shaikh Zinnat Ara Nasreen

Abstract

Menopause occurs when a woman stops menstruation permanently at the end of the reproductive life. It usually begins around the ages of 45 and 53, median age is 51. Many women experience menstrual irregularities soon before it stops. The common symptoms of menopause are that women (75%) experience vasomotor symptoms, including hot flashes, night sweats, and flushing. Headache, palpitation, and tiredness are common. Genitourinary syndrome of menopause (GSM) includes dryness of the vagina or vulvovaginal atrophy which causes sore, itching, and burning in the vagina and severe dyspareunia. Also it includes urgency, frequency, nocturia, repeated UTI, and sexual dysfunction. Mood changes like irritability, lack of concentration, loneliness, forgetfulness, insomnia, anxiety, and depression bother many women. Joint and muscle pain, backache, osteoporosis, and fracture are common. Midsection weight gain, hirsutism, hair fall, and loss of elasticity of skin are distressing symptoms. Diminished cognitive capacity, memory loss, and dementia are associated with aging, but women with premature ovarian insufficiency may experience such condition.

Keywords: vasomotor symptoms, hot flashes, VVA, GSM, osteoporosis, mood changes

1. Introduction to menopause

Menopause is a normal physiological and natural event. The WHO defined menopause as permanent cessation of menstruation due to loss of ovarian follicular activities at the end of reproductive life. Menopause before the age of 40 years is considered as premature menopause or premature ovarian insufficiency.

The average age of menopause is 51 years, which is influenced by both genetic and environmental factors. Due to increased life expectancy of women, postmenopausal years cover more than one third of the total female life span.

Though natural events of estrogen deficiency of menopause herald a variety of potential problems that can affect the quality of life, specific concerns include subjective symptoms such as vasomotor instability, i.e., hot flushes, psychological and psychomotor disorders, menstrual irregularities, vaginal dryness, genitourinary dysfunction, and osteoporosis which have implications for long-term health [1–6].

So doctors and menopausal women both are interested in and deserve an understanding of the symptoms and the basis for therapeutic recommendation aimed at relieving symptoms and reducing subsequent health risks.

IntechOpen

2. Definition

Natural menopause is recognized to have occurred after 12 consecutive months of amenorrhea, for which there is no other obvious pathological or physiological cause. Menopause occurs with the final menstrual period, which is known with certainty only in retrospect a year or more after the event. An adequate independent biological marker for the event does not exist.

The term "perimenopause" should include the time immediately prior to the menopause (when the endocrinological, biological, and clinical features approaching menopause commence) and the first year after menopause.

The term "menopausal transition" should be reserved for the time before the final menstrual period when variability in the menstrual cycle is usually increased. This term can be used synonymously with "premenopausal."

Relationship between different time periods surrounding the menopause (modified from the WHO 96238) is shown in the table below.

FMP

Stages	−5 to −4	−3	−2	−T″	+1	+2	
Terminology	Reproductive		Menopausal transition	Post	Menopause		
	Early peak	Late	Early	Late	Early late		
Perimenopause							
Duration of stage variable			Variable		1 year	4 years demise	Until
Menstrual cycles	Variable to regular	Regular	Variable cycle length > 7 days different from normal	>2 skipped cycles and an interval of amenorrhea	12 months amenorrhea	None	
Endocrine	Normal FSH	$\uparrow$ FSH	$\uparrow$ FSH		FSH		

Stages of reproductive aging workshop (STRAW) system.

3. Symptoms of menopause

3.1 Menstrual irregularities

Menstrual irregularities are a common complaint during menopause transition. Infrequent **ovulation** and anovulation lead to changes in the length of proliferative phase, and in the absence of progesterone, decline of estrogen leads to heavier and irregular menstruation. In some women scanty periods with long cycles may be the main symptom. The changes of bleeding pattern due to hormonal fluctuation usually occurs during perimenopause. The analysuisreported median age at inception of perimenopause is 47.5 years and smokers have not only early but a shorter perimenopause [2]. However, postcoital bleeding, prolonged bleeding, and postmenopausal bleeding require further investigation.

3.2 Vasomotor symptoms

Vasomotor symptoms are the main bothering and common symptoms in the early menopause. They include hot flushes, night sweats, and palpitation and are termed vasomotor symptoms because of vascular reactivity with initial prominent vasodilatation.

Hot flushes are transient periods of intense heat in the upper part of the body usually accompanied by sweating. Its exact mechanism is not known, but is believed to be due to narrowing of thermoregulatory zone of the hypothalamus with decline of estrogen level. Hot flushes and night sweats are experienced by about 40% in early transition, increasing to 60–80% in late menopausal women [3]. About 25% can be severe to cause significant distress. Sleep disturbances caused by hot flushes and sweating can lead to lethargy, poor physical functioning, and depressed mood. In about 25% of women, hot flushes may continue for over 5 years; in a small percentage of women, it may continue up to 10 years or more. In surgical menopause, vasomotor symptoms are abrupt and severe. Low body weight, lack of exercise, and smoking are risk factors for hot flushes.

Severity, frequency, and duration of hot flushes vary with menopausal status, ethnicity, age, cultural factors, and woman's perception of menopause. In many western countries and Australia, 60–80% of women experience hot flushes, while the prevalence is 20–30% in Chinese and Japanese women. In Asia 40–60% of women have hot flushes. Hot flushes have a negative impact on quality of life as well as an association with adverse morbid conditions like cardiovascular disease, osteoporosis, fragility fractures, and diabetes [4].

3.3 Mood disorders

Mood swings, anxiety, and depression are some of the psychological symptoms during menopausal change. Nearly half of women on menopause transition can get easily irritated. They become less patient with the members of the family, friends, and colleagues and often feel tired and sad. With emotional changes, they can appear nervous, stressful, and sometimes aggressive. Mood swings are due to changes in serotonin activity following estrogen decline but may also be caused by other menopausal symptoms as hot flushes and night sweats.

Anxiety in the form of nervousness, worry, or panic attacks may occur during perimenopause. Hormonal changes, vasomotor symptoms, and midlife stresses contribute to anxiety during this period. Panic disorders are associated with negative life events, impairment of activity, or physical illnesses.

Depression is more common in the menopause transition and early postmenopause than premenopausal. A number of reports indicate that there is a significant increased risk of new-onset depression in women during menopause [5]. Those who had previous episodes of depression are at a higher risk. Depression is associated with hormonal changes during this period, stressful life events, poor sleep, hot flushes, employment status, ethnicity, and cultural attitudes.

Insomnia may be seen in some women, and they are more likely to have anxiety, stress, and depressive disorders. Sleep disorders are associated with menopause transition and also related to hot flushes, other physical health problems, psychosocial problems, and medication. Sleep apnea too may occur during this period, and obese women are at a higher risk.

3.4 Genitourinary symptoms

Estrogen receptors are present abundantly in the vagina, vestibule, and trigone area of the bladder. With estrogen deficiency after menopause, many anatomical and physiological changes occur in this area, which results in GSM. Genitourinary syndrome of menopause (GSM) is the new term for vulvovaginal atrophy (VVA). In 2012, the International Society for the study of Women's Sexual Health and the North American Menopause Society introduced genitourinary syndrome of menopause as a more accurate, comprehensive, and publicly acceptable term to replace atrophy or atrophic vaginitis. The Society considered "atrophy" to be a negative term, which suggests "wasting away" and that vaginitis imply an infective or inflammatory condition. Neither the old terms encompass the urological symptoms. Furthermore, "vagina" was not regarded as a socially acceptable enough word to use in public discourse or the media (Maturitas 2014; 79–349).

Due to menopause, the withdrawal of estrogen causes dryness of the vagina, loss of elasticity and flexibility of the vagina, and damage of the vaginal epithelium. So women complain of the following:

Vaginal dryness or lack of lubrication
Dyspareunia
Postcoital soreness and bleeding (Maturitas 2014; 79–349)
Vulval/vaginal itching, soreness, burning, and discomfort
Urinary frequency, urgency, nocturia, and recurrent UTIs
Urge incontinence

On examination the vagina seems short and narrow, with the absence of rouge, and appears pale. About 20–30% of postmenopausal women have urgency and have urinary incontinence. With genital prolapse, women may suffer from recurrent urinary tract infections.

This dryness of the vagina causes decreased lubrication and sexual dysfunction [6]. The single entity of dyspareunia affects all that domains of sexual function. If not treated timely, women complain severe sexual dysfunction, which totally disrupt the conjugal life.

3.5 Osteoporosis

Accelerated osteoclastic activity and reduced osteoblastic activity and calcitonin activity due to reduced estrogen and aging process lead to osteoporosis. Osteoporosis is a systemic skeletal disease characterized by low bone mass and micro architectural deterioration of bone tissue leading to enhanced bone fragility and a consequent increase in fracture risk. Osteoporotic fracture burden is increasing worldwide. About half of women 50 and older will have an osteoporosis-related fracture in their lifetime. During the menopausal transition period, the average reduction in bone mass density (BMD) is about 10%. Approximately half of women are losing bone even more rapidly, perhaps as much as 10–20% in those 5–6 years around menopause.

Women could be asymptomatic, or they might have persistent unexplained back pain, recurrent fractures, fracture from minimal trauma, loss of height, and spinal deformities. The incidence of fractures increases, particularly of the distal radius, vertebral body, and upper femur beyond menopause. Wedge compression fractures of the spine lead to backache. Women complaining chronic back pain, bone pain, joint pain, and muscle pain must consult a doctor to exclude osteoporosis. Maintaining optimum body weight and avoiding sedentary work, bone toxic agents, too much alcohol, and smoking are the key strategies to prevent osteoporosis.

3.6 Cardiovascular disease

With the loss of cardioprotective action of estrogen by its action on lipids, endothelial function, and anti-inflammatory effect, menopausal women are more liable to get ischemic heart disease. Symptoms of coronary heart disease (CHD) in women are somewhat different from typical male type of angina, which are usually brought by exertion and relieved by rest. Women with myocardial infarction have atypical symptoms like fatigue, shortness of breath, and atypical chest pain. Many may have nonobstructive coronary heart disease (CHD); angiogram may not show typical obstruction in the coronary arteries. CHD is the commonest cause of death among postmenopausal women; the ratio of CHD in men to women becomes 1:1

after menopause. The SWAN study suggested that the protective effects of HDL might decrease during menopause [7].

3.7 Obesity

Menopause along with aging process is associated with an increased risk of obesity and a shift to an abdominal fat distribution with associated increase in health risks. Changes in body composition at menopause may be caused by the decrease in circulating estrogen. For fat distribution shifts, the relative increase in the androgen-estrogen ratio is likely to be important. Large majority of these women have an increased body mass index and waist circumference. Midsection fat distribution is pronounced during menopause and beyond. Women gaining weight especially with increased abdominal girth are prone to develop metabolic syndrome and cardiovascular disease.

But weight gain during midlife and beyond is just not due to menopausal status [8]. So women must try to maintain the optimum body weight.

3.8 Skin changes

Dry skin and wrinkling are due to the loss of subcutaneous fat and changes in composition of connective tissue. Dry hair and hair loss and increased facial hair are caused by reduction in estrogen and relative increase in male hormones. Skin becomes less elastic and wrinkling appears. Nails become brittle and nail growth becomes slow.

3.9 Joints

Osteoarthritis is commoner in females after menopause, and many epidemiological and clinical studies indicate estrogen deficiency as one of the etiological factors in addition to familial tendency, obesity, and aging. In menopausal women, the knees and hands are mostly affected.

3.10 Sarcopenia

Menopausal transition is associated with accelerated loss of fat-free mass, a decline in resting metabolic rate, and increased central body fatness. The causes of sarcopenia or loss of muscle mass are due to hormonal changes at menopause, low levels of physical activity, reduced protein intake, and increased oxidative stress.

3.11 Eyes

Postmenopausal women are at a higher risk of developing age-related macular degeneration, and association with estrogen deficiency has been suggested.

3.12 Teeth

In the menopausal woman, osteoporosis may lead to loss of the alveolar bone of the jaws, resulting in periodontal disease, loose teeth, and tooth loss. Estrogen therapy has been shown to increase the alveolar bone mass.

3.13 Memory loss

As estrogen affects cognitive function and neurotransmitters, memory loss has been noted at menopause, especially episodic memory and verbal fluency. Estrogen therapy at menopause, whether it reduces the risk of dementia and mild cognitive impairment, is a matter of debate. Women complain of bothersome memory symptoms, forgetfulness, and difficulties with word retrieval and brain fog [9].

3.14 Alzheimer disease

Alzheimer's disease (AD) is more common in postmenopausal women than in men of the same age. It is accompanied by progressive cognitive impairment and reduces the quality of life of the woman. These women have memory loss and confusion and are unable to recognize family members and friends. Often they have repetitive statements and movements and may have difficulty in getting up from a chair. Aging and other factors along with menopause are responsible, so menopause is not the direct cause of AD.

4. Key points

- The diverse symptoms associated with menopause are mainly caused by estrogen deficiency.
- Manifestations are seen in different body systems.
- Problems such as vasomotor symptoms, menstrual irregularities, joint pain, sarcopenia osteoporosis, and genitourinary disorders are troublesome and common.
- Pathologies such as osteoporosis, obesity, coronary heart disease, mood disorders, and memory problems have significant morbidity and mortality.
- Proper identification and timely optimum treatment may prevent the long-term health risks and ameliorate the symptoms of menopause and improve the quality of women's life.

Author details

Shaikh Zinnat Ara Nasreen
Department of Obstetrics and Gynaecology, ZH Shikder Women's Medical College and Hospital, Dhaka, Bangladesh

*Address all correspondence to: zinnatn@yahoo.com

References

[1] Taffe JR, Dennerstein L. Menstrual patterns leading to the final menstrual period. Menopause. 2002;**9**:32

[2] McKinlay SM, Brambilla DJ, Posner JG. The normal menopause transition. Maturitas. 1992;**14**:103

[3] Thurston EC, Joffe H. Vasomotor symptoms and menopause: Findings from the study of women's health across the nation. Obstetrics and Gynecology Clinics of North America. 2011;**38**:489

[4] Crandall CJ, Tseng CH, Crawford SL, et al. Association of menopausal vasomotor symptoms with increased bone turnover during the menopause transition. Journal of Bone and Mineral Research. 2011;**26**:840

[5] Cohen LS, Soares CN, Joffe H. Diagnosis of management of mood disorder during the menopausal transition. The American Journal of Medicine. 2005;**118**(Suppl 12B):93

[6] Sarrel PM. Ovarian hormones and vaginal blood flow; using laser Doppler velocimetry to measure effects in a clinical trial of post menopausal women. International Journal of Impotence Research. 1998;**10**(Suppl 2):S91

[7] Woodard GA, Brooks MM, Barinas-Mitchell E, et al. Lipids, menopause and early atherosclerosis in study of women's health across the Nation Heart Women. Menopause. 2011;**18**:376

[8] Sternfed B, Wang H, Quesenberry CP Jr, et al. Physical activity and changes in weight and waist circumference in midlife in midlife women: Findings from the study of women's health across the nation. American Journal of Epidemiology. 2004;**160**:912

[9] Rentz DM, Weiss BK, Jacobs EG, et al. Sex differences in episode memory in early life midlife; impact of reproductive aging. Menopause. 2017;**24**:400

Chapter 5

Endometrial Histology and Safety on Non-Oral Routes of Hormone Therapy for Perimenopausal/Early Menopausal Women: Transdermal Estrogens and Vaginal Micronized Progesterone

Manuela Cristina Russu

Abstract

The Women's Health Initiative issues, confusions, and misunderstandings regarding women's and medical staff's fears about coronary heart disease; stroke; venous thromboembolism; breast cancer; metabolic, cognitive and mood disorders; and general mortality have driven many attempts to promote other safe regimens for perimenopause/early menopause and midlife health. Perimenopause/early menopause climacteric syndrome may be safely treated with sequential transdermal/percutaneous estrogens and progestogens/vaginal progesterone or continuous transdermal estrogen plus intrauterine system medicated with progestogen/progesterone or with continuous combined transdermal estrogen-vaginal progesterone regimen, when menopause since 3 years. Endometrial safety is assessed in terms of endometrial hyperplasia and carcinoma prevention. Transvaginal sonography, hysteroscopy, and endometrial biopsy at 6/12 months ensure about secretory and atrophy/inactive endometrial aspects as markers for endometrial safety. The majority of endometrial carcinomas depicted after MHT are high grade, not estrogen dependent, developed on an atrophic endometrium. The histologic, genomic, and transcriptomic assessments with immunohistochemistry are diagnoses adjunct for cell proliferation/mitosis and apoptosis presence. Proteins, growth factors, cytokines as PAX2, PTEN and its genetic aberrations, microRNA-binding protein family (IMP, IGF-BP, progesterone dependent), bcl 2, Ki-67, K-ras, p53, p16, and steroid (estrogen and progesterone) receptors are markers for differentiation between benign hyperplasia/endometrial intraepithelial neoplasia, type 1/type 2 endometrial carcinomas, and long-term outcome.

Keywords: non-oral routes, hormone therapy, perimenopause, menopause, endometrial hyperplasia, endometrial carcinoma

IntechOpen

1. Introduction: update on the importance of the hormone treatment in perimenopausal women—non-oral routes of hormone therapy

The menopausal transition is associated with profound dynamic and critical changes of the reproductive tract, and in the hypothalamic-pituitary-ovarian axis, which have been well chronicled and matched with concomitant symptoms regarding the characteristics of menstrual cycle—the most important parameter in the new criteria of STRAW +10 (2012), which starts with the irregularities from stage-3b/-3a in the late reproductive age [1, 2], and of all other organs and tissues of the women's body, biology and psychology through this time of life. There are ethnic differences in symptoms and hormones that may reflect either basic biologic variations in hormone receptors and actions or the different social milieus that women in different ethnic groups experience [3]. The highly prevalent menopausal symptoms are sufficiently bothersome to drive almost 90% of women to seek out their healthcare provider for advice on how to cope with it. Current medical management of perimenopause should include screening for general health maintenance, avoidance of weight gain—a very important parameter for endometrial health—and a holistic approach to symptoms (**Figure 1**).

Menopausal hormone therapy (MHT) is indicated for the treatment of vasomotor symptoms and menopausal genitourinary syndrome caused by hypoestrogenism. MHT helps in the prevention of osteoporosis, colorectal cancer, type 2 diabetes mellitus, and possibly coronary heart disease (CHD), and Alzheimer's disease if started early in the perimenopause or early postmenopause—+1a/+1b (STRAW +10) in the "window of opportunity," with a positive effect on quality of life and reduction of global mortality.

The initial and quick publication of the results of Women's Health Initiative (WHI) (2002) led to confusion and fear regarding medical recommendations and women's use of MHT in conjunction with CHD, stroke, and venous thromboembolism, metabolic disorders, breast cancer, cognitive and mood disorders, and general

	Menarche						FMP (0)			
Stage	-5	-4	-3b	-3a	-2	-1	+1 a	+1b	+1c	+2
Terminology	REPRODUCTIVE				MENOPAUSAL TRANSITION		POSTMENOPAUSE			
	Early	Peak	Late		Early	Late	Early			Late
					Perimenopause					
Duration	*variable*				*variable*	1-3 years	2 years (1+1)		3-6 years	*Remaining lifespan*
PRINCIPAL CRITERIA										
Menstrual Cycle	Variable to regular	Regular	Regular	Subtle changes in Flow/ Length	*Variable Length* Persistent ≥7- day difference in length of consecutive cycles	Interval of amenorrhea of >=60 days				
SUPPORTIVE CRITERIA										
Endocrine FSH				Variable*	↑ Variable*	↑ >25 IU/L**	↑ Variable		Stabilizes	
AMH			Low	Low	Low	Low	Low		Very Low	
Inhibin B			Low	Low	Low	Low	Low		Very Low	
Antral Follicle Count			Low	Low	Low	Low	Very Low		Very Low	
DESCRIPTIVE CHARACTERISTICS										
Symptoms						Vasomotor symptoms *Likely*	Vasomotor symptoms *Most Likely*			*Increasing* symptoms of urogenital atrophy

* Blood draw on cycle days 2-5 ↑ = elevated

**Approximate expected level based on assays using current international pituitary standard[67-69]

Figure 1.
The stages of reproductive aging workshop +10 staging system for reproductive aging in women (adapted from Ref. [1]).

mortality [4]. The analyze of risks of endometrial and colon cancer proved their reduction by MHT in postmenopausal women, being proven by the reduction of colon cancer by HT in postmenopausal women.

Timing of therapy is time since menopause, being more important than women's age. When the benefits are higher than risks, as was proven by previous observational studies, animal models, and new RCT—as Kronos Early Estrogen Prevention Study, Early Versus Late Intervention Trial With Estradiol, Estrogen and Thromboembolism Risk, at near 10 years from the premature closure of both arms of WHI (2002, 2004), when on recorded the "end of an era". The personalized recommendations of MHT, or tailoring the use of MHT to appropriate candidates, with the ultimate goal of developing a personalized risk/benefit prediction model must take into account clinical and genetic factors, "patient-centered" outcomes as sense of well-being, and/or quality of life.

1.1 Non-oral versus oral route for hormone therapy administration: advantages and disadvantages

Oral HT was and still may be the most commonly used route of administration in the USA and all over the world. Evidence suggests that oral delivery may lead to some undesirable physiologic effects caused by significant gut and hepatic metabolism.

After closure of the estro-progestogen arm of the WHI (2002), some researchers admitted that not all estrogens and progestogens are alike, and alternative drugs, doses, and delivery systems may exhibit better safety profiles than CEE/MPA (with co-multiple and complex studies of the WHI), with no loss of efficacy [5, 6]. The next subchapters will present the transdermal/percutaneous route for estrogens, the vaginal route for micronized progesterone, and the intrauterine systems with levonorgestrel/progesterone for recommendation in menopause transition—early and late perimenopause and early postmenopause from the road of menopause [2]. The best regimen, formula, and dosage—the lowest efficient estrogen dose—will give the opportunity to medical staff to stratify the individual risks and to personalize the MHT indications [7].

1.1.1 Transdermal/percutaneous and nasal routes for estrogens

Transdermal/percutaneous drug delivery may mitigate some of the undesirable physiologic effects caused by significant gut and hepatic metabolism of oral HT, which still may be the most commonly used route of administration for MHT in the USA and many other countries. Active systems deliver therapeutics noninvasively across intact skin by means of an electric potential (electrotransport) [8], ensuring rapid onset and termination of action, self-administration, and attainment of therapeutic hormone levels with low daily doses, with the disadvantage of the variable intra- and interindividual percutaneous absorption and skin irritation in some patients, when women use patches.

The used estrogen is 17-β-estradiol, and women from European countries (Austria, Belgium, France, Germany, Italy, Romania, Spain, Switzerland, the Netherland, and the UK), and Canada used it during the twentieth century's last decade. It is available in multiple formulations—matrix, patches (25, 50 μg/day), and non-patches, as topical gel (hydroalcoholic gel containing 0.06% or 0.1% 17β-E2), spray, emulsion, and lotion [9] and recently in the technology of micellar nanoparticles with their unique physical and chemical properties which enable transport of substances directly into the skin [10, 11].

The pharmacokinetic and pharmacodynamic differences between oral and non-oral routes of administration give to medical staff new therapeutic perspectives for fewer health risks than oral therapy with estrogen, because only systemic therapy controls the moderate and severe climacteric syndrome, and associated to these data on must remember the large interindividual variability in the pharmacokinetics of estrogens. A dose-dependent effect explains why higher dose, longer duration, and residual endogenous estrogens are known risk factors to develop endometrial lesions and uterine bleeding with estrogens, and according to this pharmacokinetic condition, and to ovarian aging and continuous synthesis of endogenous estrogens, the actual recommendation is to use the lowest estrogen dose. The oral estrogens are converted to estrone (E1), and its conjugates, with less estrogenic activity than estradiol (E2), and the extensive metabolism of oral estrogens is inducing a higher ratio of E1 to E2 in the blood stream, which is opposite to the physiological levels in premenopausal women [12], and the formation of other metabolites from conjugated equine estrogens (CEE) used in the WHI was demonstrated to be antiestrogenic or may have unrecognized pharmacologic activity in the human body [13].

The transdermal/percutaneous and nasal administration of 17β E2 avoid the first-pass liver metabolism and the significant hepatic stimulation, without supraphysiologic concentrations in the liver. E2 is delivered directly, unmetabolized in the systemic circulation, and the estrogen doses are reduced in comparison to the oral formulation, maintaining a similar E2/E1 *ratio* to that of premenopausal women, by avoidance of gut and liver metabolism. Another peculiarity of transdermal/percutaneous route is the constant blood level of estrogens, without the peaks and troughs inherent to oral estrogens [14]. This quality is providing a more consistent blood level for the control of vasomotor symptoms and sleep disorders in perimenopause [15]. The lowest effective dose which covers treatment goals was considered to be 0.014–0.0375 mg transdermal/percutaneous 17β E2 patch, and 50 μg/day was the assessed dose in the majority of studies for sequential/cyclic regimens and 25 μg/day for continuous combined regimens.

The newest application method is the estradiol metered-dose transdermal spray (EMDTS) [16], which was proven to ensure a precise dosing, with the maximum of E2 concentration at 18–20 h after application (1 or 2 or 3 puffs), and a stable level of estradiol, estrone, and estrone sulfate on the 7th–8th day of application.

Lower HT doses generally have fewer side effects, as breast tenderness and uterine bleeding, and may have a more favorable benefit-risk *ratio* than standard doses [17]. The UK General Practice Research Database for a nested case-control study showed that the risk of stroke did not increased with low-dose transdermal estrogen (≤0.05 mg/day), but increased with oral therapies and higher transdermal doses [18]. The systemic benefits of transdermal estrogens are connected to their bioavailability and metabolic peculiarities—less pronounced effects on hepatic protein synthesis, such as markers of inflammation, coagulation, and fibrinolysis, to lower or no risk of deep vein thrombosis [19], stroke [20], and myocardial infarction, even in thrombophilic patients [21], and lower or no effects on steroid-binding proteins, but more favorable effects on triglycerides [22].

One recent, large observational cohort study of postmenopausal women (45, 112 cases hormone treated, with a mean duration of 5.5 years of HT use) made a multiple statistic comparison of clinical outcomes among users of oral and transdermal estrogen (CEE or E2) therapy, with or without progestogen, in the Women's Health Initiative Observational Study on Menopause [23], and confirmed all the benefits of non-oral estrogens and their beneficial effect on the global index events (GIE) (defined as the time to the earliest of CHD, invasive breast cancer, stroke, pulmonary embolism, colorectal cancer, endometrial cancer, hip fracture, and death from any cause) and stratified the results by duration of HT usage (mean 5.5 years), age at time of HT initiation (<60 years, 60–69 years, and ≥ 70 years), years since menopause, body mass index (BMI), and ethnicity.

The fear of breast cancer is counterbalanced by transdermal estrogens and vaginal micronized progesterone, a fact demonstrated by the figures of the large observational French study E3N Cohort, which showed a small increase in the risk of breast cancer (HR: 1.31; 95% CI: 1.15–1.48), after 5 years of use, but the risk was no longer statistically significant following discontinuation of MHT (HR: 1.15; 95% CI: 0.93–1.42) [24].

1.1.2 Low-dose vaginal estrogens

Low-dose vaginal estrogen preparations as cream, suppositories, and pessaries are recommended for long-term use in symptomatic women as required, and all topical estrogen preparations have been shown to be effective in this context. There is no requirement to combine them with systemic progestogen treatment for endometrial protection, as low-dose or ultralow-dose (10 μg vaginal 17β-estradiol tablets) [25, 26] estrogen preparations do not result in significant systemic absorption, and the risk of endometrial hyperplasia and cancer is low. After 52 weeks of such treatment, a case with hyperplasia without atypia and a case with endometrial adenocarcinoma was discovered, which was considered to be previous to the 17β-E2 vaginal treatment [25]. When the estrogen is estriol—a weak estrogen, with low potency to the estrogen nuclear receptor—the endometrial and breasts' risks are null [27].

The British Menopause Society considers that it is safe to recommend only 1-year use of vaginal estrogens, and the clinicians are advised to use the lowest effective dose for symptoms' control and to counsel women regarding this [28, 29]. A vaginal ring that delivers a large dose of estrogen to the whole body may be an option for HT in hysterectomized women; vaginal rings more often deliver low doses and are considered topical therapy.

1.1.3 Vaginal versus oral route for progesterone

The addition of a progestin (progesterone/progestogen) has only one indication: endometrial protection and endometrial safety during MHT—the prevention of hyperplasia and cancer. Progesterone, the native hormone produced by the corpus luteum during the luteal phase of the menstrual cycle, is the unique option when one seeks "physiological" hormone replacement therapy. The pure progesterone was synthesized in large amount from the plant diosgenin by the chemist Russell Marker in 1940 [30]. Depending on its chemical structure, a progestogen can either enhance (e.g. hot flushes, gonadotropin release, breast epithelial proliferation, and bone mineral density) or antagonize (e.g. endometrium, arterial wall, lipid metabolism, hepatic protein synthesis, and mood) the effects of the estrogen component [31]. Progesterone/progestogens have gene effects on estrogen receptors' synthesis downregulation and metabolic effects on rising levels of the enzyme 17-hydroxysteroid dehydrogenase, which transforms E2 to E1—sulfate, a weak estrogen—and these effects mean the arrest of endometrial glandular cell proliferation, cell differentiation, and secretory activity, and stroma decidualization. Actually, it is very well known that progestins protect the endometrium by inducing secretory transformation within the endometrial glands and stroma decidualization, and their capacity to restore to the normal endometrium without signs of differentiation or secretion is assessed after minimum 6 days and daily administration for 3–6 months in the conditions of hyperplasia [32]. These facts were assessed regarding oral compounds such as MPA, levonorgestrel, and norethisterone during the last two decades of the twentieth century, and less with vaginal/transdermal route of administration. Hyperplasia was reverted by the administration of MPA continuously for 6 weeks or cyclically for 3 months (2 weeks per month), these being the two regimens most widely used during the years 1990–2000 [33].

Available progestins—progesterone/progestogens—differ largely in their hormonal pattern, and, in addition to their progestogenic and antiestrogenic actions on the endometrium, they can exert androgenic, antiandrogenic, glucocorticoid, and/or anti-mineralocorticoid effects.

Oral progesterone (P4) formulations exist but with a very low bioavailability (<10%) because of rapid intestinal and liver metabolism. After oral administration of P4, low circulating concentrations of P4 contrast with the high concentrations of its metabolites, notably 5α-reduced metabolites which are known sources of neuropsychological effects [34], reconsidered actually for neuroprotection. The micronization of the P4 molecule provides an optimal bioavailability, which depends both on the size of the P4 particles in suspension and on the nature of the oily excipient [35]. The vaginal route for micronized P4 was proposed since many years ago [36], but the new hypothesis regarding the higher endometrial P4 levels than that obtained after intravenous administration was presented by [37], being considered an opportunity for MHT. This phenomenon of preferential uterine distribution after vaginal administration was named "first uterine pass effect" [38], or "uterine specificity of vaginal progesterone" [39]. Although the serum P4 concentration is often low or "up-physiological", the endometrium shows clear and complete secretory changes, in the majority of treated cases.

The proposed mechanisms for explanation were done after many experimental and clinical studies: direct diffusion through tissue, intracervical aspiration, absorption into the portal venous system, or lymphatic circulatory system, and countercurrent vascular exchange with diffusion from utero-vaginal veins/lymph vessels to the arteries—all these mechanisms to concur in various extents to the "uterine specificity of vaginal progesterone." Nasal administration of P4 is inducing comparative serum levels, but the endometrial secretory transformation is incomplete [40].

Previous studies showed that P4 absorption from the vagina is dependent on the formulation used and on the estrogen treatment [41]. The micronization of P4 is very important, and the oral micronized progesterone capsules were re-directed to be used vaginally [42]. Micronized P4 has a more selective effect on PRs and results in less interaction with androgenic and mineral-corticoid receptors compared with other progestogens. The previous administration of estrogens to vaginal micronized P4—100 mg/200 mg—is sustaining endometrial secretory effect compared with many other more potent progestogens. Recent evidence suggests that MHT regimens containing micronized P4 can minimize the metabolic impact and reduce the risk of thromboembolism and side effects associated with progestogens [29].

There are considerable debates about whether and at which dosage micronized P4 provides effective endometrial protection if applied orally, vaginally, or

Recommended doses of micronized progesterone for endometrial protection in MHT		
Route	**Dose**	**Safe use/month and total duration of use**
Oral	200 mg/day	12–14 days/month up to 5 years
Transdermal	—	Does not provide endometrial protection
Vaginal	Sequential 45 mg/day or continuous combined 100 mg/day	10 days/month or every other day for up to 3–5 years (off-label use)

Adapted from Ref. [44].

Table 1.
Comparison of oral and vaginal route, and dosages of P4 administration for endometrial safety.

transdermally [43]. Stute P at al. [44] are presenting the international expert panel recommendations on MHT containing micronized P4, based on their systematic review of the actions of micronized P4 on the endometrium. **Table 1** presents the comparison of daily dose, number of days imposed for endometrial protection, and time duration of safety use.

1.1.4 Medicated intrauterine systems

The medicated intrauterine systems with levonorgestrel or with P4, actually accepted by many menopause societies, are minimizing systemic progestogenic side effects by direct release of progestogen/progesterone into the endometrial cavity and directly opposing the estrogens—natural or from HT. It is presented an endometrial protection which is equivalent to that provided by systemic continuous progestogen administration, and superior to sequential progestogen regimen [45].

2. Endometrial safety on MHT: history, regimens, endometrial assessment, and endometrial histology during MHT

2.1 History

The review of climacteric symptom alleviation in the medical literature shows that the attempts are approximately 100 years old, starting with ovarian extracts, but in time it was demonstrated the ovarian responsibility for endometrial growth up to adenocarcinomas, as in ovarian transplantation [46] or in estrogen secreting ovarian tumors [47–49], cited by Van Gorp and Neven [50]. Long time it was a minimal knowledge on the real estrogen dose per day to correct the menopausal estrogen insufficiency, and on the imposed dose of progesterone to balance endometrial estrogen induced proliferation [51], for prevention of endometrial hyperplasia and cancer [52, 53]. After observational, cohort, and animal studies were designed large prospective RCTs, as it was WHI with 2 arms, closed early than it was intended initially. After a proper WHI patient reanalysis, new perspectives were discovered for the medical communities of medical staff and women.

The post-WHI analysis [54] discovered a high incidence of endometrial cancer [55], specially an increase over time in women aged 50–74 years (with an annual percentage change, in 2004–2009: 2.8%; in 2005–2009: 3.3%; and 2006–2009: 4.2%) [56], parallel to the decrease in the use of FDA-approved estrogen plus progestogen HT and parallel to the increase of endometrial hyperplasia [57], and after the increasing usage of compounded bioidentical HT (CBHT) instead of pharmacological products [58, 59], even if CBHT are not approved by the FDA, because both hormone compounds lack of standard [type (estrogen: is E2 or E3), dosage, (under dosage), and underpotency (for progesterone)] [60].

The number of cases with hyperplasia/endometrial cancer analyzed in different studies was small, fact that gives us contradictory results on endometrial safety on MHT, and there are few analyses on non-oral MHT. The largest prospective study to date on over 700,000 women, Million Women Study [61], which had done information on HT, reported a 30% reduction in risk associated with continuous regimens (based on 73 cases), but other observational studies have shown either no association or increased risks with use of continuous regimens, and some studies showing evidence of a dose-response relation with increasing duration of use (≥10 years) or increasing progestin dose. Compared with never users of HT, the risk was: reduced with last use of continuous combined preparations [RR = 0.71 (95% CI 0.56–0.90); P = 0.005].

The "European Prospective Investigation Into Cancer and Nutrition" [62] analyzed the association of various types of HT with the risk of endometrial cancer among 115,474 postmenopausal women, during 1992–2000, and after a mean follow-up period of 9 years, 601 incident cases of endometrial cancer were identified. In comparison with never users of HT, risk of endometrial cancer was increased among current users of E-only HT, with (HR = 2.52, 95% CI: 1.77–3.57), and, to a lesser extent, E + P use (HR = 1.41, 95% CI: 1.08–1.83), although risks differed according to regimen, and type of progestin constituent. The finding of a strong increased risk of endometrial cancer with estrogen-only HT, and a weaker association with combined HT supports the hypothesis that progesterone/progestogens have an attenuating effect on endometrial cancer risk.

The North American large prospective "Diet and Health" Study of National Institutes of Health-AARP (NIH-AARP) [63] among 19,131 North American postmenopausal women reporting exclusive E plus progestogen use, between whom 176 cases developed endometrial cancer (RR = 0.88; 95% CI: 0.74–1.06), and the HRs for different regimens HT showed a little increase in comparison to the previous European Study. Long-duration (≥10 years) sequential E+ P (<15 days P/month) use was positively associated with risk (RR = 1.88; 95% CI: 1.36–2.60), whereas continuous E + P use (>25 days P/month) was associated with a decreased risk (RR = 0.64; 95% CI: 0.49–0.83). The American authors' opinion is that findings support the fact that specific used categories of E+P increase the endometrial cancer risk: specifically long durations of sequential progestogens, whereas decreased endometrial cancer risk was observed for users of short-duration continuous progestogens add to estrogen.

The National Institutes of Health-AARP Diet and Health Study cohort, which did the follow-up for endometrial cancer risk after WHI's premature closure, [64] did confirm a statistical reduction of endometrial cancer risk after continuous combined oral MHT for 5.6 years (RR = 0.85; 95% CI, 0.53–1.36), with normal endometrium at entry, and including women in the highest BMI groups; this review was done because the data were not clear after immediate publication of WHI (2002, 2004).

Parallel to these data, the "European Prospective Investigation Into Cancer and Nutrition" shows a strong association of risk among women who were older, leaner, or had ever smoked cigarettes [62], and the North American studies show an increased risk for sequential E + P only among thin-to-normal weight women (BMI < 25 kg/m^2; RR = 2.53) [63]. California Teachers Study [65] reports that continuous-combined MHT was confined to thinner women (BMI < 25 kg/m^2) (P for interaction: 0.03), and among heavier women (BMI ≥ 25 kg/m^2), use of continuous-combined EPT was associated with a statistically nonsignificant reduction in risk, fact that is different from what was assumed in normal weight women. The association between endometrial cancer risk in continuous-combined MHT users to patients' BMI is correlated to women's lower endogenous estrogen levels, suggesting that menopausal hormones and obesity increase endometrial cancer through common etiologic pathways, as was recently considered that a BMI ≥ 25 kg/m^2 is increasing the rate of recurrence in patients hormonally treated for complex hyperplasia/carcinoma (P = 0.0004, OR 0.4; 95% CI: 0.3–0.6), or early stage carcinoma (P = 0.0000, OR 0.3; 95% CI: 0.2–0.6) [66] (**Figure 2**).

Healthy lifestyle index including diet, alcohol consumption, physical activity, body mass index, cigarette smoking, is recently correlated to endometrial cancer risk in Canada [67] and USA [68], and higher scores reflecting a healthier behavior of postmenopausal women are associated to reduction of endometrial cancer risk of various intensity according to the degree of type 1 cancer differentiation. Each unit increase in the HLI score was associated with 3% and 5% reductions in risk of postmenopausal endometrial cancer risk (HR 0.95; 95% CI: 0.90–0.99). The American

HT Use	Mean Duration of HT Use, years	No. of Cases	No. of Noncases	HR (95% CI)
Never		314	64,192	1.00 (referent)
Ever		287	50,607	1.44 (1.20, 1.74)
Former		83	15,633	1.16 (0.90, 1.48)
Current	2.6	196	33,657	1.72 (1.39, 2.14)
Duration of current HT use, years				
<2	1.0	40	6,918	1.67 (1.13, 2.49)
2–5	2.8	50	8,428	1.81 (1.24, 2.63)
>5	8.1	11	1,596	2.18 (1.15, 4.12)
Type of current HT				
Estrogen-only	2.6	39	4,279	2.52 (1.77, 3.57)
Estrogen plus progestin	2.5	121	24,879	1.41 (1.08, 1.83)
Tibolone	4.1	13	977	2.96 (1.67, 5.26)
Other	5.0	4	652	2.70 (0.96, 7.57)

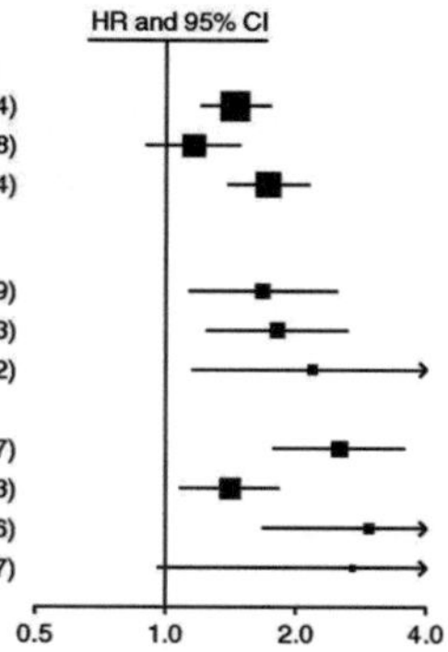

Figure 2.
Hazard ratios (HRs) for risk of endometrial carcinoma (black squares) according to use of menopausal hormone therapy (HT), by recruitment center and age, European Prospective Investigation into Cancer and Nutrition, 1992–2006. The size of each square is inversely proportional to the variance of the logarithm of the relative risk. HRs were adjusted for body mass index, parity, age at menopause, and oral contraceptive use. Bars, 95% confidence interval (CI). Adapted from Ref. [62]. Permission of Oxford Publishers.

HLI showed that after a median follow-up of 17.9 years there were 1435 endometrial cancer cases, and women in the highest quintile of the HLI score had a lower risk of overall, type I, well-differentiated, moderately differentiated, poorly differentiated, and localized endometrial cancer than those in the lowest quintile [for quintile 5 vs. quintile 1, HR = 0.61 (95% CI: 0.51, 0.72), HR = 0.60 (95% CI: 0.49, 0.72), HR = 0.66 (95% CI: 0.46, 0.96), HR = 0.69 (95% CI: 0.52, 0.90), HR = 0.49 (95% CI: 0.34, 0.72), and HR = 0.61 (95% CI: 0.50, 0.74), respectively].

2.2 Regimens of MHT: uterine bleeding on perimenopausal/menopausal hormone therapy

The chapter will discuss MHT with non-oral administrated natural estrogens which are available for perimenopausal and postmenopausal women, in comparison to oral available drugs, including contraceptive pills, among which there are some with natural estrogens, as are the estrogens in MHT. The history of MHT describes three types of MHT systemic regimens with estrogens and progesterone/progestogens for women with intact uterus, and only one systemic regimen with natural estrogens in hysterectomized women. Exogenous hormones are influencing endometrial cycle, and may also influence uterine volume, fibroid growth, polyps, endometriosis, and the development of cervical adenocarcinomas [50]. Progesterone/progestogens are mandatory for endometrial protection, as it is known since long time. Regarding endometrial safety one must discuss the characteristic of uterine bleed which appears in conjunction to the type of regimen, and the medical staff must counsel patients.

2.2.1 Sequential combined estrogen-progesterone/progestogen therapy

The sequential/cyclic administration of HT has minimum 10 days of progesterone/progestogen, more safe is 12–14 days. In this regimen both hormones are oral or non-oral administrated, or only one is on a non-oral route. If the last menstrual period occurred less than 1 year prior to starting MHT, a sequential combined regimen should be started, i.e. continuous estrogen with progesterone/progestogen for 12–14 days per month [29]. Thereby reducing the risk of endometrial hyperplasia. The patients will have a monthly withdrawal bleed with this regimen, which usually starts from the 11th day of progesterone/progestogen when this administration is for 10 days [69], and the endometrial thickness at transvaginal sonography (during the progestin administration) is higher than 4 mm at least in the first year of use [70]. Prescription of cyclic transdermal/percutaneous E2, and the sequential addition of natural progesterone or a synthetic progestogen induces artificial cycles with regular withdrawal bleeding.

2.2.2 Continuous combined estrogen-progesterone/progestogen therapy

Both hormones are administered oral or non-oral, or only one is non-oral. These regimens are increasingly used early in postmenopausal women, and the large long term Medical Research Council randomized controlled trial on HT, the Women's International Study of Long Duration Estrogen after the Menopause, and the WHI study in the USA are based on this type of oral treatment, being accepted also for women with endometrial hyperplasia without atypia. This type of regimen is discussed after a minimum 6 [69] to 12 months of sequential MHT [29] or 1 year after the last menstrual period (2 years in women with premature ovarian insufficiency). Women who wish to avoid a monthly withdrawal bleed may attempt a switch to a continuous combined regimen, which aims to give bleed-free MHT. This will minimize also the risk of endometrial hyperplasia, as it was previously discussed. There may be some erratic bleeding to begin with, but on persistence with continuous combined regimens 90% of women become bleed free.

British Menopause Society [20] has some recommendation for some special situations with uterine bleeding on continuous combined HT, as follows:

- If breakthrough bleeding occurs following the switch to continuous combined HRT and does not settle after 3–6 months, then the woman can be switched back to a sequential regimen for at least another year.

- If bleeding is heavy or erratic on a sequential regimen, the dose of progestogen can be doubled or duration increased to 21 days.

- Persistent bleeding problems beyond 6 months warrant investigation with ultrasound scan, and endometrial biopsy if clinically indicated.

2.2.3 Cyclic hormone replacement therapy using quarterly progestogen during 1 year or long cycle hormone replacement therapy

By the year 1994, Ettinger B (USA) proposed a cyclic hormone regimen with quarterly progestogen instead of monthly, aiming endometrial protection from hyperplasia and cancer, fact that was accomplished by 10 mg/day of MPA for 14 days at every 3 months [71], and with gestodene 50 μg for the last 12 days of 84 days with continuously 17β E2 in different doses—1 or 2 mg/day, with 1 year duration in the Netherlands [72]. These studies reported less bleeding episodes, with longer duration, and similar high number of hyperplasia compared to baseline assessment. In the Nordic countries this type of MHT regimen is popular, and the Scandinavian study [73] with a duration of 4 years reported partially similar results, but they used norethindrone acetate at a dose of 1 mg/day, for 10 days associated to 17β E2 2 mg per day, reduced to 1 mg day during the last 6 days of each cycle of 12 weeks. They reported a higher rate of drop-out due to bleeding vs. monthly progestogen ($P < 0.01$), and hyperplasia incidence of 5.6% vs. 1% in the monthly group ($P = 0.003$), with 1 case of atypical hyperplasia, and 1 case of endometrial adenocarcinoma. The popularity of this regimen is correlated to the 2-fold elevation of endometrial cancer risk in Finland population, and the risk reduction after cessation of the regimen [74].

Hormone	Preparation
Transdermal estrogen	17β-estradiol patch 17β-estradiol gel 17β-estradiol emulsion 17β-estradiol spray
Vaginal estrogen	17β-estradiol cream Conjugated equine estrogen cream 17β-estradiol ring 17β-estradiol tablet Estriol cream Estriol soft capsules
Vaginal progesterone	Micronized progesterone—soft capsules, gel
Transdermal progesterone/progestogens	Norethindrone acetate Levonorgoestrel
Progestin: intrauterine system	Levonorgestrel Progesterone

Table 2.
Available non-oral estrogens and progesterone/progestogens for MHT.

Besides these analyses, there is no proper study on non-oral administrated hormones, neither estrogens or progesterone/progestogen, because the Spanish study [75] assessing endometrial stability by the rate of amenorrhea and endometrial stimulation is monitoring the intermittent administration of 100 mg vaginal micronized progesterone to a patch delivering low-dose estradiol (25 μg/day). According to the Scandinavian data on hyperplasia and cancer risk [76, 77] in long cycle progesterone/progestogen regimen the bleeding pattern is not sufficient for endometrial safety, being mandatory endometrial monitoring with ultrasound and biopsies (**Table 2**).

2.2.4 Uterine bleeding on hormone therapy: is it predictive for uterine histology?

Women who start MHT from early stages of STRAW (−3 stage) may benefit from therapy with progesterone/progestogens, which balances their hormonal milieu, but starting replacement after 1 year amenorrhoea may induce the major disadvantage—the unpredictable bleeding and/or spotting, which are common in the early months of use, no matter what regimen is used. The unpredictability and persistence (in the short term) of bleeding and/or spotting is a common cause for discontinuation.

At the beginning of this century the Australian researchers [78] have presented 2 patterns for bleeding when on MHT: scheduled "withdrawal" bleeding, or unscheduled "breakthrough bleeding", usually for sequential, respectively for continuous combined regimen. Depending on the regimen, the endometrium may be proliferative, secretory, near atrophic or a mixed picture, and bleeding may occur from either an estrogen-dominated or a progestogen-dominated endometrium. When recommending continuous-combined regimen after a long duration of amenorrhea, the incidence of breakthrough bleeding is high in the first 3–6 months.

Since many years it is considered that the bleeding pattern cannot be a good predictor for endometrial histology, and safety, but it is an exception with progesterone/progestogen withdrawal bleeding in the sequential regimens, after 3 to 6 cycles of therapy, and when it is a complete secretory transformation, the bleeding may be cyclic in the last 5 days of progesterone/progestogen, or in the first 6 days of the next cycle [79]. Hyperplasia is not predicted by regular bleeding on HT, as a multicenter study suggests [80].

The variations of endometrial answers to transdermal estrogen and vaginal micronized progesterone are reduced in comparison to HT oral route, according to more stable transdermal/percutaneous estrogen serum levels, and progesterone uterine first pass. When the bleeding pattern is observed comparative to endometrial histology, the patients with proliferative histologic pattern are bleeding early than the patients with secretory transformation [81].

An Italian prospective study [82] evaluated and compared uterine bleeding in 100 early postmenopausal women (12–36 months after last mensis) on a sequential regimen with both hormones administered non-oral, *versus* the same regimen with oral natural progesterone (NP). All groups were treated with transdermal 17β-E2 50 μg/day, and the NP was 100 mg or 200 mg per day from the 14th day to the 25th day of each 28-day cycle. After 12 cycles of treatment, no significant differences were observed in endometrial thickness between groups, suggesting that all treatments are effective in balancing the estradiol effects on endometrium. Regarding bleeding control, patients in the group with sequential vaginal NP showed a higher number of episodes of regular bleeding than patients in groups with oral NP, and fewer episodes of spotting. Authors' conclusion was that transdermal estrogen combined with vaginal 100 mg micronized NP from the 14th day to the 25th day of each 28-days cycle leads to a good cycle control, and provides excellent patient satisfaction without serious side-effects. The better control of bleeding was associated with a higher treatment compliance in patients who received vaginal NP, with a larger percentage of women completing the study. The authors recommend to start treatment with the lower dose of NP (100 mg/day) to avoid the risk of amenorrhea with 200 mg/day.

An Italian study which is considered with the longest duration—3 years, has prospectively evaluated the bleeding/amenorrhea in 30 postmenopausal women treated with continuous transdermal E2 gel and every-other-day vaginal micronized progesterone in capsules [42]. They report that 4 (13%) of 30 patients withdrew from the study because of bleeding (3 for heavy bleeding and 1 for repeated spotting), and an higher incidence of amenorrhea (82%) than commonly reported (70%) with oral compounds [83].

2.3 Endometrial safety: endometrial assessment on MHT and endometrial histology on non-oral regimens of MHT

2.3.1 Endometrial safety

Endometrial safety is a grill for challenge menopausal and postmenopausal HTs, because the bleeding and the risks of hyperplasia and cancer are discussed in the 70 years of MHT history, years with many waves of increased and decreased enthusiasm on the benefits and risks of MTH. The aim of replacement and restoration of ovarian functions in postmenopausal women with estrogens and progesterone is only a modest attempt for women's health, because there are missing other molecules as testosterone, activin, inhibin, anti-Müllerian hormone (AMH) and insulin-like growth factor 1 (IGF-1), and many other connected to these, which have an immense significance on a woman's physiology, and all of them may influence endometrial actions of MHT [84].

The endometrial safety means the protection from non-invasive proliferative lesions—hyperplasia, and invasive—carcinoma.

- If the analysis of histological data is done after the criteria of the years 80′ the endometrium must be with secretory changes in the sequential regimens, and atrophy, or inactive after the continuous—combined regimens.

- If the analysis of histological data is done after the criteria of the years 90′ endometrial safety means to reduce the risk of hyperplasia and carcinoma development, in fact to down-regulate estrogen induced proliferation, with disappearance of mitosis from the endometrial glands, and stroma, or ≤2 mitoses at 1000 cells, the so-called proliferation index, or mitotic index [44].

The impact of vaginal progesterone on the endometrial safety is very important, being considered that the duration is more important than the dose [85]. After the results of the Scandinavian study regarding long cycle progestogen association to estrogen—at 3 months interval [86], which was updated in *Cochrane Database Systematic Review* [87, 88], today it is considered that it is important to combine a progesterone/progestogen with the estrogen in the beginning of the treatment, to control early endometrial growth. If one considers these Scandinavian studies, one may accept a non-opposed estrogen administration as Van Gorp and Neven recommend [50]. Minimum 10 days/month of vaginal administration provides protection in sequential regimens, in a dose of 45 mg/day at 4% in cream, or every other day in a dose of 100 mg/day for up to 3–5 years (off-label use) [44], but this aim is not accomplished with transdermal micronized progesterone [89, 90]. The daily balance of non-oral estrogen by non-oral progesterone/progestogen in continuous combined regimens is more stable than the balance of oral administration, and endometrial carcinoma risk is also reduced, as since long time ago it was reported after 8 years of use [91]. If oral and non-oral routes of progesterone/progestogen administration are proved to be less effective in treatment of atypical endometrial hyperplasia, and unable to stop most early invasive cancers, the intrauterine system with levonorgestrel 20 μg /day associated to transdermal estrogens was demonstrated to achieve these aims after 3 years administration. From 20 Belgian women, only one asymptomatic women with atypical hyperplasia at baseline at 3 years was discovered with focal residual non-atypical hyperplasia, in the presence of a thin (<4 mm) endometrium [92].

In 2002, Van Gorp and Neven [50] have published in "Maturitas" the Journal of the European Menopause and Andropause Society a review of endometrial safety on MHT. They presented a Finish study [93] on the endometrial safety after short term HT (12 months) regarding percutaneous estradiol-gel delivering E2 1.0 mg/day, or patch (delivering E2 50 pg/day) in a sequential regimen with oral dydrogesterone 10 mg/day for first 12 days of the cycle. The endometrial biopsies—collected during the 9th to 12th days of the progestogen days in both groups did not revealed any hyperplasia, or any estrogenic effect.

2.3.2 Endometrial assessment on menopausal hormone therapy

MHT must be assessed when women start therapy, with an annual follow-up or when there is a minimal suspicion of endometrial abnormality regarding bleeding, or when it is an abnormality at transvaginal scan by endometrial biopsy, with Pipelle Cornier suction curette, Kevorkian or Vabra curette, or by fractional curettage—endometrium and endocervix, or by out-patient hysteroscopy. Hysteroscopy permits to avoid the loss of an isolated focus of endometrial cancer, atypical hyperplasia or polyp which easily can be missed by blind sampling procedures [70]. On another hand hysteroscopy is prone to depict the changes of endometrial surface, vessels, which are very much discussed by the Australian gynecologists and pathologist in connection to bleeding pattern on MRT [78].

Besides some inconvenients which will be discussed in the next subchapter, the endometrial sample obtained with Pipelle Cornier suction curette has been shown to be as accurate as conventional dilation and curettage in the diagnosis of endometrial pathology in premenopausal and postmenopausal women [94]. The amount of endometrial tissue is very little, sometimes much less than that demanded by pathologists unused to such biopsies, but when the microscopy is corroborated to ultrasound, the medical staff can be reassured of safety [94].

Double layer endometrial thickness is usually measured at the thickest part in the longitudinal plane, by scanning from cornua to cornua. The poorly echogenic layer surrounding the highly echogenic endometrium is not included in the measurement. Endometrial thickness is evaluated to determine the mean of three measurements and excluding the possible endometrial fluid from the measurement. One must take into account in elder patients with atrophic endometrium after MHT that the fluid may be blood, even the patients do not bleed. In oral and non-oral MHT the endometrial thickness has an initial increase—more important after sequential regimens, with a consistent decrease at 36 months when on continuous combined regimens, so the endometrium becomes significantly thinner than at baseline. These data are controverted by the previously presented prospective Italian study, which after 12 cycles of non-oral sequential treatment discovered no significant differences in endometrial thickness between groups, suggesting that all treatments are effective in balancing the effects of percutaneous E2 on endometrium [82].

The prospective Italian study on continuous-combined non-oral MHT [42] revealed a smaller increase of the endometrial thickness comparative to that reported by a similar North American oral regimen; the baseline-to-endpoint increases in endometrial thickness were 7.8 ± 3.8 mm, and 1.8 ± 3.2 mm, respectively [95] versus the Italian data, where the mean endometrial thickness increase was only 0.7 mm, after 6 months treatment, and endometrial atrophy was registered after 3 years (end of study), in all cases that completed the study [twenty-three (76.7%) women from 30 healthy cases in natural menopause]. The British study [96] revealed a continuous increase of endometrial thickness from baseline [3.3 (1.7)] mm to the mean of 5.3 (3.3) mm by 24 weeks ($P < 0.001$), and of 5.5 (2.8) mm after 48 weeks, with continuous combined transdermal E2 1.1 mg/day plus 4 mg/day NP cream, ($P < 0.001$), being a non-significant increase from 24th to 48th weeks, but the increase was more important when it was inadequate endometrial opposition (4.7 mm vs. 7.6 mm respectively, $P < 0.001$). These results and the histological aspects of proliferative endometrium with inadequate progesterone opposition after 48 weeks HT—which will be analyzed in next subchapter, sustain the actual recommendation to avoid transdermal natural progesterone.

2.3.3 Endometrial histology with non-oral MHT

Endometrial histological assessment is a very important part of the continuing follow up of women taking MHT. There are few studies on endometrial histology after MHT with both hormones administered non-orally in comparison to oral route.

Table 3 is listing such studies, which were published after WHI, with some North American studies before the year 2000; the studied estrogens and progestogens were transdermal administered, and the soft capsules of micronized progesterone were vaginally administered. Because it is the rule of baseline endometrial assessment, the studies are comparing the histology at pre, and post-treatment, or in some of them to oral MHT. The endometrial biopsy is done before treatment, and between 9th and 14th days of treatment cycle, to evaluate the progesterone/progestogen effect (similar to cases on oral MHT), in the sequential regimens. The endometrial specimen is collected after 6 months, no matter which day, in continuous-combined MHT regimens.

Endometrial safety is assessed in terms of prevention of estrogen-induced hyperplasia. Progesterone supplementation may cover the objective of endometrial protection from benign hyperplasia from the STRAW—3 stage (2012), or when it is

Authors/study group, year Duration of use	Type and dose of estrogen	Type and dose of progestegen/ progesterone	Hyperplasia, type 1/2 cancer P value (authors conclusions/ commments)
Archer DF, Furst K, et al., 1999 [97] 3, 6, 9, and 12 months after initiation of treatment	Continuous combined estradiol 50 μg/day	Norethindrone acetate 140, 250, or 400 μg/day	0.8% (1 of 123), 1% (1 of 98), 1.1% (1 of 89) ($P < 0.001$)
Ylikorkala O, Rozenberg S, 2000 [98] 12 months	Continuous combined or sequential E2 50 μg/day	Continuous combined Trd NETA: 170 μg/ day or sequential Trd NETA: 350 μg/day, or sequential oral NETA 1 mg/day or sequential DYD 20 mg/day	2 cases of simple hyperplasia were reported (1 in each low-dose progestogen group)
Shulman LP, Yankov V, Uhl K, 2002 [99] 12 months	Continuous combined, once a week patch E2 0.045 mg/day	LNG mg/day of 0.015; 0.030; and 0.040	No hyperplasia
Sturdee DW, van de Weijer P, von Holst T, 2002 [100] 12 months	Sequential: 3 groups 1. patches of 15 cm^2 (50 μg/day E2 for 2 wks, followed 50 μg/day E2–10 μg/day LNGl for 2 wks) 2. 22.5 cm^2 (75 μg/dy E2 for 2 weeks followed by 75 μg/day E2–15 μg/day LNG for 2 wks) 3. 30 cm^2 (100 μg/day E2 for 2 wks followed by 100 μg/day E2–20 μg/day LNG for 2 wks)		Endometrial protection for all groups
Dando TM, Perry CM (2004) [101] 17 beta-E2/LNG transdermal system 12 months, RCT	Continuous combined, 2 groups with once a week Patch 17 β estradiol:+ LNG 4.4/1.39 or 4.4/2.74/day or 4.5/3.75 mg/day		No hyperplasia
Cicinelli E, de Ziegler D, Colafiglio G, et al., 2005 [42] 3 years montoring	Continuous combined 17 β estradiol gel, 1.5 mg/day	Micronized progesterone, soft capsules 100 mg every-other-day (or at 48 h) (vaginal)	No hyperplasia Atrophy: 100%
Vashisht A, Wadsworth F, Carey A, Carey B, Studd J, 2005 [96] 48 weeks (54 cases, only 41 completed the study)	Continuous combined oestradiol 1 mg/day transdermal daily	Natural progesterone cream 40 mg/day (transdermal)	10 (27%) endometrial proliferation, 2 (5%) complex hyperplasia, 1 with (mild) atypia, and 1 without atypia
Samsioe G, Dvorak V, Genazzani AR, et al., Estalis 25/125 Study Group, 2007 [102] 96 weeks	Continuous combined estradiol matrix 25 μg/day	NETA 125 μg/day	No hyperplasia No cancer
Russu M, Terzea D, Hudiță D, 2009 [103] 24 months monitoring	Sequential HT 1. Group oral: 2 mg/d E2 valerate (E2V) 21 days, E2V plus CYP 10 days 2. Group oral: 2 mg/d -mcr E2 14 days, 2 mg/d mcrE2 plus DYD 14 days 3. Group mixed: 17β E2 patch (25 μg/d 21 days) plus oral MPA (10 mg/5 mg/day) last 12 days 4. Group fully non-oral: 1 g/d 17β E2 gel 28 days plus 200 mg/d vaginal micronized VMP last 12 days		1 case with simple hyperplasia without atypia after 24 months, on transdermal estrogen +5 mg MPA (incidence 1/43 cases) is inside the oncological safety (2 cases/100 women year) No carcinoma

Authors/study group, year Duration of use	Type and dose of estrogen	Type and dose of progestegen/ progesterone	Hyperplasia, type 1/2 cancer P value (authors conclusions/ commments)
Fernandez-Munga L, Hermenegildo C, Tarin JJ, Garcia-Perez M-A, Cano A, 2012 [75] 12 months	Intermittent (twice a week) Estradiol patch 25 μg/day	Intermittent (twice a week) 100 mg micronized progesterone (vaginal)	No apparent endometrial stimulation

E2, estradiol; LNG, levonorgestrel; NETA, norethisteron enanthate; E2V, estradiol valerate; CYP, cyproterone acetate; DYD, dydrogesterone; VMP, vaginal micronized progesterone.

Table 3.
Studies on endometrial histology and safety after non-oral routes of MHT.

the onset of menstrual cycle irregularities, which may have hyperplasia as histologic substrate.

The effects of hormones are appreciated on the architecture and cytological aspects of the epithelium, glands, stroma, and vessels. Mitoses are considered for estrogens proliferative effect, and subnuclear glycogen accumulation, and intraluminal secretions for high grade progesterone effects, or the cytoplasmic vacuolisation, for low grade progesterone secretory change [104, 105]. When progesterone regulation effect is not possible to be assessed with accuracy, the degree of proliferation suppression—mild, moderate, strong is a surrogate for evaluation, as it was done in the Romanian analysis [103].

There are many pathologists involved in endometrial assessment on/after MHT in Europe, USA, Canada, South Africa. **Table 4** presents an adaption of endometrial changes on MHT according to International Society of Gynecological Pathologists (2019) [112, 113], WHO (2014) cited by [123], British Society for Gynecological Endoscopy (2014) [120], FIGO (2009, 2012) cited by [119]. Deligdish [104], Feeley and Wells [94] present very understandable the endometrial effects of MHT, including a wide spectrum of morphologic features, known since long time on oral MHT, and less on non-oral routes, which are. Recently discussed by Owings and Quick [105]. For simplicity of understanding, **Table 4** contains the classification of endometrial histology changes, with special attention to the hyperplasia [WHO, 1994, with 4 types updated by WHO, 2014, cited by [123], which was recommended for use by the Royal College of Obstetricians and Gynecologists (RCOG), and the British Society for Gynecological Endoscopy (BSGE) [120], with only 2 categories, as it is mentioned in the table, and it was discussed at the beginning of the subchapter].

The first three types (unassessable, inactive, atrophic) may impose some problems to the pathologist, because there is a small amount of tissue—obtained with Pipelle suction curette, and the British pathologists Feeley and Wells [94] appreciate that this condition can be associated to thin, regular endometrium at hysteroscopy, or with an endometrial thickness not exceeding 7 mm, at sonography [108], and though the pathologist can therefore be reassured that where the endometrial cavity has been entered and little or no endometrial tissue is obtained, there is very little likelihood of important endometrial pathology to be present. The assessment of secretory endometrium may be confused by artifacts of fragments disruption, which may induce focal changes of glandular tortuosity and crowding. The diagnosis of low grade cytological atypia is very difficult to be appreciated [94]. In a progesterone/progestogen rich environment, nuclei of premalignant glands tend to diminish in size, and acquire a rather bland chromatin pattern, which makes them

Unassessable

- No tissue identified
- Tissue insufficient for diagnosis
- No endometrium identified
- Endometrial tissue insufficient for diagnosis

Inactive

- Narrow tubular glands lined with cuboidal epithelium

Atrophic

- Cystically dilated glands lined by single layer of inactive, flattened epithelial cells

Proliferative

- Presence of epithelial mitoses

Secretory

- Epithelial cytoplasmic vacuolation—subnuclear or supranuclear
- Glandular luminal secretion in mid-phase and late phase

Pseudo-decidual change

- Typical stromal decidual change associated with inactive or weakly secretory glands, induced by progestogen

Benign hyperplasia (BH), Mutter [106] or endometrial hyperplasia without atypia (WHO, 2014), which covers formerly named simple and complex hyperplasia without atypia (WHO, 1994)

- Simple hyperplasia without atypia:
- Dilated glands with increased nuclear stratification of lining epithelium and increased stromal mitoses.
- No risk of malignancy
- Complex hyperplasia without atypia
- Crowded and irregular branched glands
- Low risk of malignancy

Atypical endometrial hyperplasia (WHO, 2000), or endometrial intraepithelial neoplasia (EIN)—[106, 107]

- Atypical epithelial cells; high risk of malignancy

Carcinoma (endometrioid type, non-endometrioid type)

Adapted from WHO (2014) which updated WHO (1994); [106, 107, 121].

Table 4.
Classification and associated features of histological examination of the Pipelle endometrial biopsy.

appear less "atypical". Paradoxically, the nuclei of normal glands become enlarged and rounded—features associated with atypia [109].

The endometrium aspect depends on the regimen; it may be proliferative, secretory, near atrophic, inactive, or a mixed picture-mixed proliferative and secretory endometrium including crowded and hyperplastic glands, alternating with an edematous, hyperplastic, or decidualized stroma, sometimes with thickened or thrombosed blood vessels.

Most endometrial biopsies from women on sequential MHT show weak secretory features. Approximately 15% show proliferative activity, although this figure may be less if more than 9 days of progesterone/progestogen is given per cycle. A small proportion are revealing an inactive or atrophic endometrium. Up to 50% of biopsies in cases on continuous combined HT contain minimal tissue for pathological analysis: this correlates well with an atrophic endometrium with no appreciable pathology. Of the 50% with more substantial material, approximately one half presents endometrial atrophy, and one half are showing weak secretory features [94]. The Romanian analysis shows that after complete non-oral route of HT, the proliferative rate and secretory changes were more frequent in the first year, and atrophy was after oral HT. The analysis regarding endometrial stroma has revealed two important aspects to be discussed:

- the increase of stroma the fibroblast-fibrocytic proliferation, and the reduction of fibrosis in all treated cases, indirectly the maintenance of the stroma volume (an important criteria when on discuss about EIN, with volume percentage of stroma <55%). This change makes the difference between normal cycling endometrium and the iatrogenic one.

- the increase of the granulocyte inflammatory reaction, which is like a pseudo-decidualisation, not a sign of endometritis, which need to discover the presence of periglandular plasma cells, and leukocytes. In the natural menstrual cycle the presence in endometrial stroma of the leukocytes infiltration is normal in the premenstrual phase, when starts the decline of estrogen and progesterone, aspect which is rarely discovered, but it is discussed also by Deligdish [104] in sequential regimens, as a probable result of the iatrogenic hormones withdrawal.

3. Endometrial hyperplasia and endometrial cancer risks in MHT: immunohistochemistry for biomarkers of endometrial transcriptome in MHT

3.1 Endometrial hyperplasia and cancer

Endometrial cancer is the fourth cancer in women from developed countries [110], and actually there are 2 types of endometrial cancer, with different natural history, carcinogenesis and evolution.

According to the molecular mechanisms, to the dualistic model of endometrial cancer development, first time described by Bokhman [111], the last classification at the Endometrial Cancer Workshop sponsored by the International Society of Gynecological Pathologists in 2016 [112], and the most recent discussion of the International Society of Gynecological Pathologists in 2019 [113] describes low grade and high grade endometrial cancers, both types being discussed to have MHT in perimenopause and late postmenopausal stages of women's life.

- low grade or type 1 or endometrioid endometrial or the "indolent" cancer, which is estrogen dependent, has "atypical endometrial hyperplasia", as precursor (23% cases progress to endometrioid adenocarcinoma), a monoclonal lesion, with microsatellite instability, and *ras* and *PTEN* mutations [106, 107, 109, 114, 115], and PTEN gene loss in up to 65% cases with EIN and in 85% cases with endometrioid carcinoma [116], with estrogen and progesterone receptors at immunohistochemistry analysis [110] discovered more frequent in white, Caucasian women.

- high grade endometrial carcinomas or type 2 are represented by previous FIGO grade 3 endometrioid carcinoma, serous endometrial carcinoma, clear cells endometrial carcinoma, undifferentiated/dedifferentiated carcinoma, and carcinosarcoma. They are non-estrogen dependent, more aggressive, with atrophia or with a polyp rather than hyperplasia as precursor, and they are non-responsive to progestins [32]. They contain *p53* mutations and abnormal accumulation of p53 protein, and absence of ERs, PRs [117, 118]. In cases with serous endometrial carcinoma the estrogen level is low, but SHBG is high, women are 6 years elder, with lower BMI than the cases with type 1.

The FIGO grading 1, 2 and 3 of endometrioid endometrial adenocarcinomas are actually nominated only in two grades, as follows: former grade 1 and 2 are the actual "low" grade endometrioid endometrial carcinomas, and former grade 3 is the actual "high grade" [119], although FIGO, the ACOG, and the College of American Pathologists are considering this grading as standard.

Hyperplasia and endometrioid endometrial cancer risk is associated to excess levels of estrogen, or to non-balanced/non-opposed estrogens by progesterone/progestogens-proved by PEPI trial (1996) [122], after the well-known paper of Kurman et al. [32], and recently reconfirmed by the "European Prospective Investigation Into Cancer and Nutrition" [62]. Mutter [106, 109] is describing benign hyperplasia—with low risk for malignancy, type that was discovered in the studies listed in **Table 3** and "Endometrial Intraepithelial Neoplasia" (EIN) the precursor for the endometrioid endometrial/type 1 cancer.

The terminology of "Endometrial Intraepithelial Neoplasia" (EIN) [109, 116] was previously termed in the World Health Organization system (1994) as atypical endometrial hyperplasia — simple, and complex. There is no direct concordance of WHO to EIN categories because the two strategies employ different criteria that are often nonequivalent [123]. On must remember that approximately 50% of women diagnosed with atypical hyperplasia have concurrent carcinoma [124].

The WHO (1994) system largely relies on relatively fixed notions of how atypical endometrial cells appear, whereas an EIN criterion combines crowded architecture and a relative change in cytology in the high-risk category.

"Endometrial Intraepithelial Carcinoma" (EIC) [125] is considered as precursor for high grade/type 2 endometrial cancer, and it represents malignant transformation of atrophic surface endometrium, discovered in 89% of cases. "Endometrial intraepithelial neoplasia" should never be confused with "endometrial intraepithelial carcinoma", which refers clearly to type 2 endometrial cancer, usually named as serous carcinoma, and is driven by a p53 mutation. Awareness of these 2 entities and their histologic features is critical for avoiding misclassification [109, 118].

The data regarding endometrial hyperplasia/cancer on or after non-oral route of MHT are few, but generally they may be comparable to those on oral drugs. The Finnish Cancer Registry [74], which evaluated cancer risk from 1995 to 2007 recorded 1364 type 1 and 38 type 2 endometrial cancers by the end of 2006, and the study analyzed duration and type of regimen, route and type of progestogen: oral/non oral sequential (10–14 days once a month—"monthly sequential" or every three months—"long-cycle"), or continuous combined (E2 patch or gel plus NETA or LNG), or E2 transdermal + LNG-releasing intrauterine device system (LNG-IUS).

- For use of <5 years, the OR for sequential EPT was 0.67 (95% CI: 0.52–0.86), for continuous E2+ P was 0.45 (CI: 0.27–0.73), and for E2 plus LNG-IUS = 0.39, CI: (0.17–0.88).

- A decreased risk persisted for the use of continuous E2+ P and E2 plus LNG-IUS of up to 10 years.

The conclusion of the Finnish study was that the use of a continuous rather than a sequential E2-progestogen regimen decreases the risk of endometrial cancer, whereas the route of administration or type of progestin does not differ in terms of endometrial cancer risk.

A recent North American study [126] revealed that compared with non-MHT users, cases who reported using E+ P Therapy had lowered all-cause (HR = 0.65, 95% CI = 0.43–0.99) and endometrial cancer-specific mortality (HR = 0.51, 95% CI = 0.26–0.98), study which can be added to a previous study from Sweden [127], which investigated tumor grade and depth of myometrial invasion, and 5-year relative survival in postmenopausal endometrial cancer patients. In this analysis, ever use of any MHT entailed lower risks of having moderately and poorly differentiated tumors. The lowest OD for poorly differentiated tumors were seen for ever users of cyclically combined estrogen-progestin [OR = 0.23 (95% CI: 0.07–0.73)]. Ever users of any form of MHT, particularly medium potency MHT users, had significantly lower risks for tumors with deep myometrial invasion, and adjusted estimated relative excess HRs revealed significantly improved survival for ever users of any form of MHT [RER = 0.40 (95% CI: 0.16–0.97)]; in particular ever users of any form of oestrogens [RER = 0.38 (95% CI: 0.15–0.99)]. The authors' conclusions were that MHT ever used induces a more favorable tumor characteristics, less aggressive and with better patients' survival.

3.2 Immunohistochemistry for hyperplasia and endometrial cancer risk on MHT: endometrial transcriptome and biomarkers

Endometrium is a tissue with strong capacities of renewal/remodeling for cell proliferation/new tissue formation, differentiation, apoptosis, angiogenesis which are highly regulated by ovarian steroids, and various locally expressed gene products, and with the presence of regenerative endometrial stem cells with their special capacities, which are maintained in menopause. The role and qualities of endometrial stroma in EIN, and cancer progression are very important, and the mechanisms of E and P4 in promoting proliferation on one side, secretory activity and differention on the other side are connected to the steroid receptors presence, and to the transformation of endometrial transcriptome, because of gene or epigenetic changes by hypermethylation of DNA and histones, with overexpression or underexpression of genes that encodes the proteins necessary for successful proliferation, apoptosis, angiogenesis, and fight against endometrial epithelial glands and stroma atypia The reported "hyperplasia" and no endometrial cancer from **Table 3** is not sufficient for the outcome prediction for long time. Molecular genetic researches related to hereditary predisposition (as Lynch syndrome, and Cowden syndrome) and to epigenetic changes are now used for uterine structures too, and endometrial transcriptome is more and more understood.

There are histological biomarkers for endometrial transcriptome assessment: estrogen (ER), progesterone (PR) receptors, membrane estrogen and progesterone receptors, and their polymorphism; enzymes involved in E2 metabolism to E1, and other molecules as bcl-2, p53, PAX-2, PTEN, VGEF, and microRNA (miRNA) can help to make the differences in the outcome of each patient. The proliferative activity induced by estrogen increases the risk for errors in transcription (microsatellite instability, K-ras mutation, PTEN gene mutations), which are essential for carcinogenesis [128]. Microsatellite instability (MSI) is a condition manifested by damaged DNA because of defects in normal DNA repair process; it induces progression of hyperplasia with atypia to endometrioid endometrial carcinoma—reported to be 20–45% in such cases, and 0–11% in type 2 endometrial carcinoma.

Estrogen may operate through "classical" genomic pathways (*via* nuclear ERs) or non-genomic pathways (ERs in plasma membrane/cytoplasm or other receptors/adaptors). Approximately 10% of the patients with type 1 endometrial cancer show gene defects promoting carcinogenesis; one representative example is hereditary non-polyposis colon cancer (HNPCC), known as Lynch syndrome [129] when the lifetime risk for endometrial cancer is 40–60% [130].

miRNAs are short (19–25 nucleotides) naturally-occurring, non-coding RNA molecules that base-pair with the 3′ untranslated region of target miRNAs. miRNAs have emerged as key regulators of gene expression, a single miRNA can target and potentially silence several hundred genes, and their involvement in aging by modulating the presence of steroid receptors, and other molecules in endometrial disorders, as are EIN, and both types of endometrial cancer. Recent studies have identified miRNAs regulated by estrogens in human endometrial stromal cells [131], fact discussed because E2 levels decline in postmenopause, and are various age-associated disorders.

Endometrial transcriptome analysis using techniques of immnohistochemistry may reveal women's risk to progesterone/progestin resistance and progression to EIN by measuring PRA and PRB; high expression of PRA and PRB suggesting decreased risk of persistence/progression to EIN, and the decrease of PRB is strongly associated to progression to EIN. No association was found with PTEN, and PTEN mutations, Pax-2, and Bcl-2, insulin like-growth factor II, with complex hyperplasia [132].

4. Conclusions: future perspectives for middle aged women treated for perimenopausal symptoms

The discussed non-oral routes of MHT, meaning the transdermal/percutaneous route for estrogens, the vaginal route for micronized progesterone, and intrauterine system for proges-terone/progestogen are an update safe option for women with intact uterus, when the recommendation for MHT is during the "window of opportunity". The technology of obtaining these drugs/system will help medical staff and middle aged women to have a better quality of life, and less morbidity and mortality. The risk of endometrial proliferative lesions as hyperplasia and carcinoma is reduced in comparison to non-user women, and their prognosis is better comparative to non-users regarding tumor aggression and women's survival. Endometrial transcriptome and new biomarkers highlight priority areas for future research, such as increasing the diagnostic reproductibility of endometrial hyperplasia-benign, and EIN and to improve the discrimination between EIN and carcinoma, and identifying new biomarkers to stratify risks or serve as indicators of response to clinical treatment.

Conflict of interest

Nothing to disclaim.

Thanks

I thank Romanian patients who trust on my recommendations regarding non oral routes for MHT, when the majority used the oral route.

Author details

Manuela Cristina Russu
"Dr. I. Cantacuzino" Discipline of Obstetrics and Gynecology, "Carol Davila" University of Medicine and Pharmacy, Bucharest, Romania

*Address all correspondence to: manuela_russu@yahoo.com

References

[1] Harlow DS, Gass M, Hall EJ, Lobo R, Maki P, Rebar WR, et al. For the STRAW +10. Executive summary of the stages of reproductive aging workshop +10. Addressing the unfinished agenda of staging reproductive aging. The Journal of Clinical Endocrinology & Metabolism. 2012;**97**(2):1159-1168. DOI: 10.1210/jc.2011-3362

[2] Santoro N. Perimenopause: From research to practice. Journal of Women's Health. 2016;**25**(4):332-339. DOI: 10.1089/jwh.2015.5556

[3] Santoro N, Chervenak JL. The menopause transition. Endocrinology and Metabolism Clinics of North America. 2004;**33**(4):627-636

[4] Lobo AR. Where are we 10 years after the Women's Health Initiative? The Journal of Clinical Endocrinology & Metabolism. 2013;**98**(5):1771-1780

[5] Nelson HD. Commonly used types of postmenopausal estrogen for treatment of hot flashes: Scientific review. JAMA. 2004;**291**(13):1610-1620

[6] Carroll N. A review of transdermal nonpatch estrogen therapy for the management of menopausal symptoms. Journal of Women's Health. 2010;**19**(1):47-55. DOI: 10.1089/jwh.2008.120

[7] Manson JE. The role of personalized medicine in identifying appropriate candidates for menopausal estrogen therapy. Metabolism. 2013;**62**(Suppl 1): S15-S19. DOI: 10.1016/j.metabol.2012.08.015

[8] Henzi MR. Optimizing delivery of therapeutics: Percutaneous technologies. Bratislavské Lekárske Listy. 2002;**103**(4-5):144-151

[9] Egras AM, Umland EM. The role of transdermal estrogen sprays and estradiol topical emulsion in the management of menopause-associated vasomotor symptoms. International Journal of General Medicine. 2010;**3**:147-151

[10] Simon JA, ESTRASORB Study Group. Estradiol in micellar nanoparticles: The efficacy and safety of a novel transdermal drug-delivery technology in the management of moderate to severe vasomotor symptoms. Menopause. 2006;**13**(2):222-231

[11] Valenzuela P, Simon JA. Nanoparticle delivery for transdermal HRT. Nanomedicine. 2012;**8**(Suppl 1): S83-S89. DOI: 10.1016/j.nano.2012.05.008

[12] Gleason CE, Carlsson CM, Johnson S, Atwood C, Asthana S. Clinical pharmacology and differential cognitive efficacy of estrogen preparation. Annals of the New York Academy of Sciences. 2005;**1052**:93-115

[13] Campagnoli C, Ambroggio S, Biglia N, Sismondi P. Conjugated estrogens and breast cancer risk. Gynecological Endocrinology. 1999;**13**(Suppl 6):13-19

[14] Kopper WN, Gudman J, Thompson JD. Transdermal hormone therapy in postmenopausal women: A review of metabolic effects and drug delivery technologies. Drug Design, Development and Therapy. 2008;**2**:193-202

[15] Cintron D, Lipford M, Larrea-Mantilla L, Spencer-Bonilla G, Lloyd R, Gionfriddo MR, et al. Efficacy of menopausal hormone therapy on sleep quality: Systematic review and meta-analysis. Endocrine. 2017;**55**(3):702-711

[16] Fait T, Fialova A, Pastor Z. The use of estradiol metered-dose transdermal spray in clinical practice. Climacteric. 2018 Dec;**21**(6):549-553. DOI: 10.1080/13697137.2018.1504916

[17] The North American Menopause Society. The 2012 hormone therapy position statement of the North American menopause society. Menopause. 2012;**19**(3):257-271. DOI: 10.1097/gme.0b013e31824b970a

[18] Renoux C, Dell'aniello S, Garbe E, Suissa S. Transdermal and oral hormone replacement therapy and the risk of stroke: A nested case control study. BMJ. 2010;**340**:c2519

[19] Scarabin PY, Oger E, Plu-Bureau G, on behalf of the Estrogen and THrombo Embolism Risk (ESTHER) Study Group. Differential association of oral and transdermal oestrogen-replacement therapy with venous thromboembolism risk. Lancet. 2003;**362**:428-432

[20] Canonico M, Carcaillon L, Plu-Bureau G, Oger E, Singh-Manoux A, Tubert-Bitter P, et al. Postmenopausal hormone therapy and risk of stroke impact of the route of estrogen administration and type of progestogen. Stroke. 2016;**47**:1734-1741. DOI: 10.1161/STOKEAHA.116.01.3052

[21] Canonico M, Plu-Bureau G, Lowe GD, Scarabin PY. Hormone replacement therapy and risk of venous thromboembolism in postmenopausal women: Systematic review and meta-analysis. BMJ. 2008;**336**:1227-1231

[22] Goodman PM. Are all estrogens created equal? A review of oral vs. transdermal therapy. Journal of Women's Health. 2012;**21**(2):161-169. DOI: 10.1089/jwh.2011.2839

[23] Crandal JC, Hovey MK, Andrews C, Cantly AJ, Stefanick M, Shufelt C, et al. Comparison of clinical outcomes among users of oral and transdermal estrogen therapy in the women's health initiative observational study. Menopause. 2017;**24**(10):1145-1153. DOI: 10.1097/GME:0000000000000899

[24] Fournier A, Mesrine S, Dossus L, Boutron-Ruault MC, Clavel-Chapelon F, Chabbert-Buffet N. Risk of breast cancer after stopping menopausal hormone therapy in the E3N cohort. Breast Cancer Research and Treatment. 2014;**145**:535-543. DOI: 10.1007/s10549-014-2934-6

[25] Simon J, Nachtigall L, Ulrich LG, Eugster-Hausmann M, Gut R. Endometrial safety of ultra-low-dose estradiol vaginal tablets. Obstetrics and Gynecology. 2010;**116**(4):876-883. DOI: 10.1097/AOG.0b013e3181f386bb

[26] Ulrich L, Naessen T, Elia D, Goldstein JA, Eugster-Hausmann M. Vag-1748 trial investigation-endometrial safety of ultra-low-dose Vagifem 10 microg in postmenopausal women with vaginal atrophy. Climacteric. 2010;**13**(3):228-237. DOI: 10.3109/13697137.2010.481058

[27] Russu M, Mubarak N, Marin JA, Hudiță D. Quality of life improvement after vaginal treatment of urogenital atrophy symptoms in postmenopause. "Securing a healthy future to day". In: Proceedings of the 8th European Congress on Menopause (EMAS), London, UK, May, 16-20, 2009

[28] Panay N, Hamoda H, Arya R, Savvas M, on behalf of The British Menopause Society and Women's Health Concern—The. British Menopause Society & Women's Health Concern recommendations on hormone replacement therapy. The Menopause International. 2013;**19**(2):59, 2013-68. DOI: 10.1177/1754045313489645

[29] Hamoda H, Panay N, Arya R, Savvas M. The British Menopause Society & Women's Health Concern 2016 recommendations on hormone replacement therapy in menopausal women. PostReproductive Health. 2016;**22**(4):165-183. DOI: 10.1177/2053369116680501

[30] Loose DS, Stancel GM. Estrogens and progestins. In: Brunton LL, editor. Godman & Gilman's the Pharmacological Basis of Therapeutics. 11th ed. New York, NY: McGraw-Hill; 2006. pp. 1541-1571

[31] Wiegratz I, Kuhl H. Progestogen therapies: Differences in clinical effects? Trends in Endocrinology and Metabolism. 2004;**15**(6):277-285. DOI: 10.1016/j.tem.2004.06.006

[32] Kurman RJ, Kaminski PF, Norris HJ. The behavior of endometrial hyperplasia. A long-term study of untreated hyperplasia in 170 patients. Cancer. 1985;**56**:403-412

[33] Figueroa Casas PR, Ettiger B, Delgado E, Jaykin A, Vieder C. Reversal by medical treatment of endometrial hyperplasia caused by estrogen replacement therapy. Menopause. 2001;**8**(6):420-423

[34] Nahoul K, Dehennin L, Scholler R. Radioimmunoassay of plasma progesterone after oral administration of micronized progesterone. Journal of Steroid Biochemistry. 1987;**26**:241-249

[35] Hargrove JT, Maxson WS, Wentz AC. Absorption of oral progesterone is influenced by vehicle and particle size. American Journal of Obstetrics and Gynecology. 1989;**161**:948-951

[36] Price JH, Ismail H, Gorwill RH, Sarda IR. Effect of the suppository base on progesterone delivery from the vagina. Fertility and Sterility. 1983;**39**:490-493

[37] Cicinelli E, de Ziegler D. New hypotheses transvaginal progesterone: Evidence for a new functional 'portal system' flowing from the vagina to the uterus. Human Reproduction Update. 1999;**5**(4):365-372

[38] de Ziegler D. Hormonal control of endometrial receptivity. Human Reproduction. 1995;**10**:4-7

[39] Cicinelli E, Schonauer LM, Galantino P, Matteo MG, Cassetta R, Pinto V. Mechanisms of uterine specificity of vaginal progesterone. Human Reproduction. 2000; **15**(Suppl. 1):159-165

[40] Cicinelli E, Cignarelli M, Resta L, Scorcia P, Petruzzi D, Santoro G. Effects of the repetitive administration of progesterone by nasal spray in postmenopausal women. Fertility and Sterility. 1993;**60**:1020-1024

[41] Villanueva B, Casper RF, SCC Y. Intravaginal administration of progesterone: Enhanced absorption after estrogentreatment. Fertility and Sterility. 1981;**35**:433-437

[42] Cicinelli E, de Ziegler D, Alfonso R, Nicoletti R, Bellavia M, Colafiglio G. Endometrial effects, bleeding control, and compliance with a new postmenopausal hormone therapy regimen based on transdermal estradiol gel, and every-other-day vaginal progesterone in capsules: A 3-year pilot study. Fertility and Sterility. 2005;**83**:1859-1863

[43] Ruan X, Mueck AO. Systemic progesterone therapy—Oral, vaginal, injections and even transdermal? Maturitas. 2014;**79**:248-255

[44] Stute P, Neulen J, Wildt L. The impact of micronized progesterone on the endometrium: A systematic review. Climacteric. 2016;**7137**:1-13

[45] Somboonporn W, Panna S, Temtanakitpaisan T, Kaewrudee S, Soontrapa S. Effects of the levonorgestrel releasing intrauterine system plus estrogen therapy in perimenopausal and postmenopausal women. Systematic review and meta-analysis. Menopause. 2011;**18**(10):1060-1066

[46] Knauer E. Die ovarien transplantation. Expreimentelle Studie

Arch Gynaek. 1900;**60**:322, cited by Van Gorp T, 2002 [49]

[47] Murray WS. Ovarian secretion and tumor incidence. Science. 1927;**66**: 600-601, cited by Van Gorp T, 2002

[48] Dockerty MB, Massey E. Malignant lesions of the uterus associated with estrogen-producing ovarian tumors. American Journal of Obstetrics and Gynecology. 1951;**61**:147-150, cited by Van Gorp T, 2002

[49] Lilienfield AM, Johnson EA. The age distribution in female breast and genital cancers. Cancer. 1955;**8**:875-881

[50] Van Gorp T, Neven P. Endometrial safety of hormone replacement therapy: Review of literature. Maturitas. 2002;**42**:93-104

[51] Kelly RM, Baker WH. Progesterone for endometrial cancer. New England Journal of Medicine. 1961;**246**:216-220

[52] Gusberg SB. Precursors of corpus carcinoma-estrogens and adenomatous hyperplasia. American Journal of Obstetrics and Gynecology. 1947;**54**:905-907

[53] Jensen EI, Oestergaard E. Clinical studies concerning the relationship of estrogens to the development of cancer of the corpus uteri. American Journal of Obstetrics and Gynecology. 1954;**67**:1094-1102

[54] Constantine GD, Kessler G, Graham S, Goldstein SR. Increased incidence of endometrial cancer following the WHI: An assessment of risk factors. Journal of Women's Health. 2019;**28**(2):237-243. DOI: 10.1089/jwh.2018.6956

[55] American Cancer Society Endometrial cancer causes, risk factors, and prevention. Available at: https://www.cancer.org/content/dam/CRC/PDF/Public/8610.00.pdf. [Accessed: 27 November 2017]

[56] Wartko P, Sherman ME, Yang HP, Felix AS, Brinton LA, Trabert B. Recent changes in endometrial cancer trends among menopausal-age U.S. women. Cancer Epidemiology. 2013;**37**:374-377

[57] Dezman VL, Gersak MZ, Gersak K. Two case of atypical endometrial hyperplasia associated with "bioidentical" hormone replacement therapy: IGCS-0084 Uterine Cancer, including Sarcoma. International Journal of Gynecological Cancer. 2015;**25**(Suppl 1):71

[58] Eden JA, Hacker NF, Fortune M. Three cases of endometrial cancer associated with "bioidentical" hormone replacement therapy. The Medical Journal of Australia. 2007;**187**:244-245

[59] Gass ML, Stuenkel CA, Utian WH, LaCroix A, Liu JH, Shifren JL. Use of compounded hormone therapy in the United States: Report of the North American Menopause Society survey. Menopause. 2015;**22**:1276-1284

[60] American College of Obstetricians and Gynecologists Committee on Gynecologic Practice, American Society for Reproductive Medicine Practice Committee. Compounded bioidentical menopausal hormone therapy. Fertility and Sterility. 2012;**98**:308-312

[61] Beral V, Bull D, Reeves G. Million women study C. Endometrial cancer and hormone-replacement therapy in the million women study. Lancet. 2005;**365**(9470):1543-1551

[62] Allen NE, Tsilidis KK, Key TJ, Dossus L, Kaaks T, Riboli E, et al. Menopausal hormone therapy and risk of endometrial carcinoma among postmenopausal women in the European Prospective Investigation Into Cancer and Nutrition. American Journal of Epidemiology. 2010;**172**(12): 1394-1403. DOI: 10.1093/aje/kwq300

[63] Trabert B, Wentzensen N, Yang HP, Sherman ME, Hollenbeck AR,

Park Y, et al. Is estrogen plus progestin menopausal hormone therapy safe with respect to endometrial cancer risk? International Journal of Cancer. 2013;**132**(2):417-426. DOI: 10.1002/ijc.27623

[64] Chlebowski RT, Anderson GL, Sarto GE, Aragaki AK, Haque R, Runowicz CD. Continuous combined estrogen plus progestin and endometrial cancer: The women's health initiative randomized trial. Journal of the National Cancer Institute. 2016;**108**(3):1-10

[65] Razavi P, Pike CM, Horn-Ross P, Templeman C, Bernstein L, Ursin G. Long-term postmenopausal hormone therapy and endometrial cancer. Cancer Epidemiology, Biomarkers & Prevention. 2010;**19**(2):475. DOI: 10.1158/1055-9965.EPI-09-0712

[66] Li M, Guo T, Cui R, Feng Y, Bai H, Zhang Z. Weight control is vital for patients with early-stage endometrial cancer or complex atypical hyperplasia who have received progestin therapy to spare fertility: A systematic review and meta-analysis. Cancer Management and Research. 2019;**11**:4005-4021. DOI: 10.2147/CMAR.S194607

[67] Arthur R, Kirsh VA, Kreiger N, Rohan T. A healthy lifestyle index and its association with risk of breast, endometrial, and ovarian cancer among Canadian women. Cancer Causes & Control. 2018;**29**(6):485-493. DOI: 10.1007/s10552-018-1032-1

[68] Arthur R, Brasky TM, Crane TE, Felix AS, Kaunitz AM, Shadvab AH, et al. Associations of a healthy lifestyle index with the risks of endometrial and ovarian cancer among women in the women's health initiative study. American Journal of Epidemiology. 2019;**188**(2):261-273. DOI: 10.1093/aje/kwy249

[69] Sturdee DW, Barlow HD, Ulrich L, Gydesen H, Wells M, Campbell JM, et al. Is the timing of withdrawal bleeding a guide to endometrial safety during sequential oestrogen-progestogen replacement therapy? The Lancet. 1994;**344**:979-982. DOI: 10.1016/S0140-6736 (94)91640-3

[70] Stovall TG, Solomon SK, Ling FW. Endometrial sampling prior to hysterectomy. Obstetrics & Gynecology. 1989;**73**(3, Part 1):405-409

[71] Ettinger B, Selby J, Citron JT, Vangessel A, Ettinger VM, Hendrickson MR. Cyclic hormone replacement therapy using quarterly progestin. Obstetrics and Gynecology. 1994;**83**:693-700

[72] Boerrigter PJ, van de Weiner PH, Baak JP, Fox H, Haspels AA, Kenemabs P. Endometrial response in estrogen replacement therapy quarterly combined with a progestogen. Maturitas. 1996;**24**(1-2):63-71

[73] Bjarnason K, Certin A, Lindgren R, Weber T. Adverse endometrial effects during long cycle hormone replacement therapy. Scandinavian Long Cycle Study Group. Maturitas. 1999;**32**(3):161-170

[74] Jaakkola S, Lyytinen H, Dyba T, Ylikorkala O, Pukkala E. Endometrial cancer associated with various forms of postmenopausal hormone therapy: A case control study. International Journal of Cancer. 2011;**128**(7):1644-1651. DOI: 10.1002/ijc.25762

[75] Fernandez-Munga L, Hermenegildo C, Tarin JJ, Garcia-Perez M-A, Cano A. Endometrial response to concurrent treatment with vaginal progesterone and transdermal estradiol. Climacteric. 2012;**15**(5):455-459

[76] Pukkala E, Tulenheimo-Silfvast A, Leminen A. Incidence of cancer among women using long versus monthly cycle hormonal replacement therapy, Finland

1994-1997. Cancer Causes & Control. 2001;**12**:111-115

[77] Pukkala E, Rautalahti M. Cancer in Finland. Cancer Society of Finland; 2013. ISBN: 978-952-5815-16-0

[78] Thomas MA, Hickeys M, Fraser SI. Disturbances of endometrial bleeding with hormone replacement therapy. Human Reproduction. 2000; **15**(Suppl. 3):7-17

[79] Padwick ML, Pryse-Davies J, Whitehead MI. A simple method for determining the optimal dose of progestin in postmenopausal women receiving estrogens. New England Journal of Medicine. 1989;**1**:163-164

[80] Sturdee DW, Ulrich L, Barlow HD, Campbell JM, Vessey PM, Nielsen B, et al. The endometrial response to sequential and continuous combined destrogen-progestogen replacement therapy. BMJ. 2005;**107**(11):1392-1400. DOI: 10.1111/j.1471-0528.2000.tb11654.x

[81] Whitehead MI, Hillard TC, Crook D. The role and use of progestogens. Obstetrics & Gynecology. 1990;**75**(4 (suppl)):59S-79S

[82] Di Carlo C, Tommaselli GA, Gargano V, Savoia F, Bifulco G, Nappi C. Transdermal estradiol and oral or vaginal natural progesterone: Bleeding patterns. Climacteric. 2010;**13**(5): 442-446. DOI: 10.3109/13697137.2010.490605

[83] Archer DF, Pickar JH, Bottiglioni F. Bleeding patterns in postmenopausal women taking continuous combined or sequential regimens of conjugated estrogens with medroxyprogesterone acetate. Obstetrics and Gynecology. 1994;**83**:686-692

[84] Agarwal S, Alzahrani FA, Ahmed A. Hormone replacement therapy: Would it be possible to replicate a functional ovary? International Journal of Molecular Sciences. 2018;**19**(10), pii: E3160. DOI: 10.3390/ijms19103160

[85] Archer D. The effect of the duration of progestin use on the occurrence of endometrial cancer in postmenopausal women. Menopause. 2001;**8**(4):245-251

[86] Cerin A, Heldaas K, Moeller B. Adverse endometrial effects of long-cycle estrogen and progestogen replacement therapy. The Scandinavian Long-Cycle Study Group. New England Journal of Medicine. 1996;**334**:668-669

[87] Furness S, Roberts H, Marjoribanks J, Lethaby A, Hickey M, Farquar C. Hormone therapy in postmenopausal women and risk of endometrial hyperplasia. Cochrane Database of Systematic Reviews. 2009;**15**(2):CD000402. DOI: 10.1002/14651858.CD000402.pub3

[88] Furness S, Roberts H, Marjoribanks J, Lethaby A. Hormone therapy in postmenopausal women and risk of endometrial hyperplasia. Cochrane Database of Systematic Reviews. 2012;**15**(8):CD000402. DOI: 10.1002/14651858.CD000402.pub4

[89] Leonetti HB, Landes J, Steinberg D, Anasti JN. Transdermal progesterone cream as an alternative progestin in hormone therapy. Alternative Therapies in Health and Medicine. 2005;**11**:36-38

[90] Wren BG. Transdermal progesterone creams for postmenopausal women: More hype than hope. Medical Journal of Australia. 2005;**182**(5):237-239

[91] Leather AT, Savvas M, Studd JW. Endometrial histology and bleeding patterns after 8 years of continuous combined estrogen and progestogen therapy in postmenopausal women. Obstetrics and Gynecology. 1991;**78**:1008-1010

[92] Widemeersch D, Janssens D, Pylyser K, De Wever N, Verbeek G, Dhont M, et al. Management of patients with non-atypical and atypical endometrial hyperplasia with a levonorgestrel-releasing intrauterine system: Long-term follow-up. Maturitas. 2007;**57**(2):210-213. DOI: 10.1016/j.maturitas.2006.12.004

[93] Hirvonen E, Cacciatore B, Wahlström TT, Rita H, Wilén-Rosenqvist G. Effects of transdermal oestrogen therapy in postmenopausal women: A comparative study of an E2 gel and an E2 delivering patch. British Journal of Obstetrics and Gynaecology. 1997;**104**(S16):21-31

[94] Feeley KM, Wells M. Hormone replacement therapy and the endometrium. BMJ. 2001;**54**(6): 435-440. DOI: 10.1136/jcp.54.6.435

[95] Davies GC, Huster WJ, Shen W, Mitlak B, Plouffe L Jr, Cohen FJ, et al. Endometrial response to raloxifene compared with placebo, cyclical hormone replacement therapy, and unopposed estrogen in postmenopausal women. Menopause. 1999;**6**:188-195

[96] Vashisht A, Wadsworth F, Carey A, Carey B, Studd J. Bleeding profiles and effects on the endometrium for women using a novel combination of transdermal oestradiol and natural progesterone cream as part of a continuous combined hormone replacement regime. BJOG. 2005;**112**:1402-1406

[97] Archer DF, Furst K, Tipping D, Dain MP, Vandepol C. A randomized comparison of continuous combined transdermal delivery of estradiol-norethindrone acetate and estradiol alone for menopause. CombiPatch Study Group. Obstetrics & Gynecology. 1999;**94**:498-503

[98] Ylikorkala O, Rozenberg S. Efficacy and tolerability of fully transdermal hormone replacement in sequential or continuous therapy at two doses of progestogen in postmenopausal women. Maturitas. 2000;**37**(2):83-93

[99] Shulman LP, Yankov V, Uhl K. Safety and efficacy of a continuous once-a-week 17beta-estradiol/levonorgestrel transdermal system and its effects on vasomotor symptoms and endometrial safety in postmenopausal women: The results of two multicenter, double-blind, randomized, controlled trials. Menopause. 2002;**9**(3):195-207

[100] Sturdee DW, van de Weijer P, von Holst T. Endometrial safety of a transdermal sequential estradiol-levonorgestrel combination. Climacteric. 2002;**5**(2):170-177

[101] Dando TM, Perry CM. 17 beta-estradiol/levonorgestrel transdermal system. Treatments in Endocrinology. 2004;**3**(5):319-324

[102] Samsioe G, Dvorak V, Genazzani AR, Mueck AO, Arguinzoniz M, et al. One-year endometrial safety evaluation of a continuous combined transdermal matrix patch delivering low-dose estradiol-norethisterone acetate in postmenopausal women. Maturitas. 2007;**57**(2):171-181

[103] Russu M, Terzea D, Hudiță D. Endometrial histology and safety after a novel regimen with transdermal estrogen and vaginal micronized progesteron. Two years of monitoring. Maturitas. 2009;**63**(Supplement 1) Abstracts Book ISSN 0378-5122., "Securing a healthy future to day" to The 8th European Congress on Menopause (EMAS), London, UK, 16-20 May 2009

[104] Deligdish L. Hormonal pathology of the endometrium. Modern Pathology. 2000;**13**:285-294

[105] Owings RA, Quick CM. Endometrial intraepithelial neoplasia.

Archives of Pathology & Laboratory Medicine. 2014;**138**:484-491

[106] Mutter GL. Endometrial intraepithelial neoplasia (EIN): Will it bring order to chaos? The Endometrial Collaborative Group. Gynecologic Oncology. 2000;**76**:287-290

[107] Dietel M. The histological diagnosis of endometrial hyperplasia. Is there a need to simplify? Virchows Archiv. 2001;**439**(5):604-608

[108] Piegsa K, Calder A, Davis JA, McKay-Hart D, Wells M, Bryden F. Endometrial status in post-menopausal women on long-term continuous combined hormone replacement therapy (Kliofem). A comparative study of endometrial biopsy, outpatient hysteroscopy and transvaginal ultrasound. European Journal of Obstetrics, Gynecology, and Reproductive Biology. 1997;**72**:175-180

[109] Mutter GL. Diagnosis of premalignant endometrial disease. Journal of Clinical Pathology. 2002;**55**(5):326-331

[110] Silverberg GS, Kurman RJ, Nogales F, Mutter GL, Kubik-Huck A, Tavassoli AF. Epithelial tumors and related lesions, Pathology and Genetics of Tumors of the Breast and Female Organs, Devilee P, Tavassoli AF, IARC Press, Lyon, France, 2003

[111] Bokhman JV. Two pathogenetic types of endometrial carcinoma. Gynecologic Oncology. 1983;**15**:10-17

[112] Murali R, Davidson B, Fadare O, Carlson JA, Crum CP, Gilks CB, et al. High-grade endometrial carcinomas: Morphologic and immunohistochemical features, diagnostic challenges and recommendations. International Journal of Gynecologic Pathology. 2019;**38**(Suppl 1):S40-S63. DOI: 10.1097/PGP.0000000000000491

[113] Rabban JT, Gilks CB, Malpica A, Matias-Guiu X, Mittal K, Mutter GL, et al. Issues in the differential diagnosis of uterine low-grade endometrioid carcinoma, including mixed endometrial carcinomas: Recommendations from the international society of gynecological pathologists. International Journal of Gynecologic Pathology. 2019;**38**(Suppl 1):S25-S39. DOI: 10.1097/PGP.0000000000000512

[114] Levine RL, Cargile CB, Blazes MS, van Rees B, Kurman RJ, Ellenson LH. *PTEN* mutations and microsatellite instability in complex atypical hyperplasia, a precursor lesion to uterine endometrioid carcinoma. Cancer Research. 1998;**58**:3524-3528

[115] Mutter GL. PTEN, a protean tumor suppressor. The American Journal of Pathology. 2001;**158**:1895-1898

[116] Mutter GL, Zaino RJ, Robboy SJ, et al. Benign endometrial hyperplasia sequence and endometrial intraepithelial neoplasia. International Journal of Gynecological Pathology. 2007;**26**(2):103-114

[117] Zheng W, Khurana R, Felix JC, et al. p53 immunostaining as a significant adjunct diagnostic method for uterine surface carcinoma. The American Journal of Surgical Pathology. 1998;**22**:163-173

[118] Sherman ME. Theories of endometrial carcinogenesis: A multidisciplinary approach. Modern Pathology. 2000;**13**:295-308

[119] Soslow RA, Tornos C, Park KJ, Malpica A, Matias-Guiu X, Oliva E, et al. Endometrial carcinoma diagnosis: Use of FIGO grading and genomic subcategories in clinical practice: Recommendations of the International Society of Gynecological Pathologists. International Journal of Gynecologic Pathology.

2019;**38**(Suppl 1):S64-S74. DOI: 10.1097/PGP.0000000000000518

[120] Royal College of Obstetricians and Gynecologists, British Society for Gynecological Endoscopy—Management of Endometrial Hyperplasia, Green-Top Guideline No 67. 2016

[121] Wells M, Sturdee DW, Barlow DH, Ulrich LG, O'Brien K, Campbell MJ, et al. Effect on endometrium of long term treatment with continuous combined oestrogen-progestogen replacement therapy: Follow up study. British Medical Journal. 2002;**325**(7358):239

[122] The Writing Group for the PEPI Trial. Effects of hormone replacement therapy on endometrial histology in postmenopausal women. The Postmenopausal Estrogen/Progestin Interventions (PEPI) Trial. The Writing Group for the PEPI Trial. JAMA. 1996;**275**(5):370-375

[123] Salman MC, Usubutun A, Boynukalin K, Yuce K. Comparison of WHO and endometrial intraepithelial neoplasia classifications in predicting the presence of coexistent malignancy in endometrial hyperplasia. Journal of Gynecologic Oncology. 2010;**21**(2):97-101

[124] Lacey JV Jr, Chia VM. Endometrial hyperplasia and the risk of progression to carcinoma. Maturitas. 2009;**63**(1):39-44. DOI: 10.1016/j.maturitas.2009.02.005

[125] Ambros RA, Sherman ME, Zahn CM, Bitterman P, Kurman RJ. Endometrial intraepithelial carcinoma: A distinctive lesion specifically associated with tumors displaying serous differentiation. Human Pathology. 1995;**26**:1260-1267

[126] Felix SA, Arem H, Trabert B, Gierach LG, Park Y, Pfeiffer MR, et al. Menopausal hormone therapy and mortality among endometrial cancer patients in the NIH-AARP Diet and Health Study. Cancer Causes Control. 2015;**26**(8):1055-1061. DOI: 10.1007/s10552-0598-0

[127] Orgėas CC, Hall P, Wedrėn S, Dickman PW, Czene K. The influence of menopausal hormone therapy on tumour characteristics and survival in endometrial cancer patients. European Journal of Cancer. 2009;**45**(17): 3064-3073. DOI: 10.1016/j.ejca.2009.05.012

[128] Samarnthai N, Hall K, Yeh T. Molecular profiling of endometrial malignancies. Obstetrics and Gynecology International. 2010, Article ID 162363, 16 pages. DOI: 10.1155/2010/162363

[129] Chen LM, Yang KY, Little SE, Cheung MK, Caughey AB. Gynecologic cancer prevention in Lynch syndrome/hereditary nonpolyposis colorectal cancer families. Obstetrics and Gynecology. 2007;**110**:18-25

[130] Tinelli A, Vergara D, Martignago R, Leo G, Tinelli R. Hormonal carcinogenesis and socio-biological development factors in endometrial cancer: A clinical review. Acta Obstetricia et Gynecologica. 2008;**87**:11011113

[131] Klinge CM. Estrogen regulation of microRNA expression. Current Genomics. 2009;**10**(3):169-183

[132] Upson K, Allison K, Reed S, Jordan C, Newton K, Swisher E, et al. Biomarkers of progestin therapy resistance and endometrial hyperplasia progression. American Journal of Obstetrics and Gynecology. 2012;**207**(1):36e1-36e8

Chapter 6

The Role of Hormone Replacement Therapy in the Treatment of Menopausal Symptoms in Patients Diagnosed with Gynecologic Cancer

Hasan Çilgin

Abstract

The incidence of most cancers increases with age, especially from middle age onward, so today cancer can be considered an age-related disease. One of the keys to healthy and successful aging is reducing the advent of serious disabilities caused by diseases related to aging. One of the cornerstones of anti-aging is hormone replacement therapy to treat age-related diseases caused by sex hormone deficiency in women. However, there are many studies that question the relationship between hormone replacement therapies with cancer recurrence. Hormone replacement therapy (HRT) has the potential to affect both quality of life and survival in menopausal women. Although data in the literature is controversial, many clinicians remain reluctant to write HRT for gynecologic cancer patients due to fear of relapse but HRT does not appear to be associated with an increased risk of relapse in ovarian and endometrial cancer survivors, especially when used for a short period of time.

Keywords: endometrial cancer, gynecologic cancers, hormone replacement therapy, ovarian cancer, cervical cancer

1. Introduction

Menopause is defined by the World Health Organization (WHO) as the complete disappearance of cyclic menstruation over a period of 12 months due to a reduction in the production of estrogen and progesterone hormones from a woman's ovaries [1]. Menopause can be defined by more concrete values in laboratory tests. According to the findings of amenorrhea and hypestrogenemia studies, serum FSH levels above 40 IU/L were defined. Subjectively, menopause can also be diagnosed by vasomotor symptoms, such as hot flashes. The permanent cessation of menstrual periods can occur naturally or can be induced by surgery, chemotherapy or radiation, leading to estrogen deficiency and loss of reproductive function [2]. Symptoms are more pronounced with a sudden drop in circulating estrogen levels. These symptoms are severe in premature ovarian failure and surgical menopause. Natural menopause is often seen between the ages of 45 and

55, but its onset varies from woman to woman. The average age of natural menopause in our country (Turkey) is 47 [3].

A menopausal statement can disrupt a woman's personal and social life. Vasomotor symptoms (e.g., hot flashes and night sweats) are the most common symptoms and can be treated very effectively with estrogen-based hormone therapy. The decision to use estrogen (usually only hormone therapy or hormone replacement therapy or HT) treatment involves balancing potential benefits with potential risks. A woman who desires HRT and has an intact uterus must also receive progestogen with the estrogen to protect her uterus from endometrial hyperplasia or malignancy. It is assumed that if a woman has had a hysterectomy that she no longer needs a progestin. However, progesterone is different, as it can provide symptom relief from sleep disturbance and mood instability, and there is increasing evidence to support its offering protection to breast tissue [4].

The relationship between early surgical menopause and poor cognitive outcomes has been demonstrated. Increased risk of cognitive impairment especially in patients undergoing oophorectomy at a young age revealed that this relationship is age-related [5].

Furthermore, cancer treatment often accelerates menopause and then affects quality of life. Postmenopausal women are at increased risk for vaginal dryness, dyspareunia, urogenital atrophy and sexual dysfunction. Hormone replacement therapy (HRT) has been proven to be highly effective in alleviating menopausal symptoms, such as hot flashes, night sweats, dyspareunia, sexual disorders and insomnia, as well as preventing osteoporosis. Life satisfaction and social functioning can be improved by overcoming menopausal symptoms and increasing resistance to age-related pathologies.

The number of menopausal women will also increase as the population ages. Accurate estimation of the postmenopausal population is an important point for health care providers to consider, as the incidence of all cancers increases with aging. If life satisfaction, social functioning and psychological resources are enhanced by increasing resistance to against age-related pathologies, the experience of aging can be improved.

To clarify the possible effective management of menopausal symptoms, the main evidence in the literature was analyzed to investigate the role of hormone replacement therapy in patients affected by endometrial, ovarian or cervical cancer.

2. Endometrial cancer

A number of clinical trials have reported that HRT does not increase the risk of recurrence of endometrial cancer (EC) even after treatment [6, 7]. In contrast, studies' showing that estrogen exposure is associated with an increase in mitosis of endometrial cells, placing them in a specific molecular configuration sensitive to DNA damage [8].

The most common gynecological cancer, endometrial cancer is seen in the postmenopausal period, but 25% of diagnosed patients are premenopausal with approximately 2.5–14.4% of the patients less than 40 years old [9].

As a result, a large number of women will be exposed to the sudden iatrogenic onset of postmenopausal morbidity, consisting of standard abdominal hysterectomy and bilateral oophorectomy procedures. In addition, surgery-induced menopausal symptoms tend to be more severe than those caused by normal menopause, and in these patients, surgery is usually followed by chemotherapy or radiotherapy [10]. Since EC is typically diagnosed with a good prognosis in the early stage of the disease, relieving these symptoms is an important issue in terms of quality of life after treatment [11].

The endometrioid EC type is associated with estrogen exposure and endometrial hyperplasia. The role of estrogens in providing relapse after hysterectomy for EC is less clear and controversial. Since it does not increase recurrence, there are a number of current clinical studies that report HRT should be considered even after EC therapy [12]. For relief of menopause-related vasomotor symptoms (VMS), systemic usage of HRT with either (1) conventional estrogens/progestogens or (2) conjugated estrogens/bazedoxifene is the most effective regime. Currently, method 2 conjugated estrogens, with a selective estrogen receptor modulator such as bazedoxifene, is a very popular replacement of progestin. This method is useful for protection of the endometrium.

Although these finding were based on retrospective or cohort controlled study results, HRT use does not seem to increase the risk of EC recurrence. Creasman et al. reported a retrospective study of 47 cases of stage I endometrial cancer patients treated with via the oral or vaginal route using conjugated estrogen (0.625 or 1.25 mg/dl). HRT was initiated within 15 months (range 0–81 months) of the median interval after cancer treatment and patients were followed up for 32 months (range 6–84 months) after the onset of HRT. In the control group, 174 patients who began treatment at the same time were compared. No difference was observed between the groups in terms of prognostic aspects. Only one recurrence (2.1%) was observed in the estrogen-treated group and 26 recurrences (14.9%) were observed in the control group. The recurrent patient in the HRT group had been treated with estrogen only for 3 months and had discontinued HRT use 18 months before relapse. Disease-free survival (DFS) and overall survival (OS) were significantly longer in the estrogen-treated group [13].

A retrospective paired cohort study was conducted with 75 women being treated for stages I–III EC who received an average of 83 months of HRT (conjugated equine estrogen-oral, 0.625 mg/dl with or without medroxyprogesterone acetate-oral, 2.5 mg/dl). These women were then compared with matched controls who received an average of 69 months of treatment. The study revealed lower recurrence rate (1 vs. 14% in the control group) and significantly longer DFS ($P = 0.006$) in the HRT group [14].

A total of 50 patients with stage I or stage II EC who had combined HRT (0.625 mg conjugated equine estrogen plus continuous oral daily regimen and 2.5 mg medroxyprogesterone acetate) of 4–8 weeks postoperatively were compared to 52 patients for control purposes. In the first prospective paired cohort study, no recurrence was observed in the HRT group but a relapse was observed in the control group [12].

A retrospective case-control study was conducted with 44 clinical stage I patients (defined as grade 1 or 2 tumors), using oral estrogens (0.625 or 1.25 mg/dl) with or without combined progesterone. The study revealed no metastases to lymph nodes or other organs [15].

Serous papillary and clear cell carcinomas, which are mostly seen in postmenopausal women and constitute approximately 8% of all ECs, have poor prognosis even if they are caught at an early stage. Since they do not have estrogen and progesterone receptors, it is not thought that they are not stimulated when HRT is used after surgical treatment. A safe recommendation cannot be raised because no study has addressed the use of HRT after treatment in all of the above histological subtypes of EC. As for uterine sarcomas, endometrial stromal sarcomas are considered estrogen-dependent because they express estrogen and progesterone receptors, and the application of HRT in these sarcomas should be avoided [16].

Although it is mainly based on retrospective, case or cohort controlled studies based on various biases, the use of HRT, in women with stage I and/or II EC, the risk of relapse was demonstrated with data that did not increase. Selecting healthier and younger women to explain the protective effect of HRT on recurrence in survivors of EC may eliminate this publication bias.

Although it is based on retrospective or cohort-controlled studies, nowadays, a number of clinical studies have reported that HRT should be considered even after treatment of endometrial cancer (EC) without increasing the risk of recurrence [17].

Although the results related to EC do not completely exclude the possibility of increasing the risk of recurrence, they argue that HRT does not matter the magnitude of such a risk. The positive effect of HRT on quality of life outweighs the unfounded risk of recurrence. Additional well-designed RCTs are needed for the definite recommendations including the factors that may be related to recurrence such as characteristics and treatment of cancer, different types of HRT, the disease-free interval before the onset of HRT, and the duration of HRT use. To determine the best therapeutic option between new hormones and non-hormonal regimens every EC survivor dealing with HRT must be informed of the available data and analyzed in a personalized way.

3. Ovarian cancer

Worldwide, among patients diagnosed with gynecological malignancies, ovarian cancer is the leading cause of death. Most women affected are postmenopausal, but some are younger. Menopausal symptoms in the iatrogenic group are generally more pronounced than those following naturally occurring menopause and affect quality of life and health outcomes [18, 19].

After the treatment of a serious disease such as ovarian cancer, more attention should be paid to the women's quality of life. Presently, the WHO, Europe, and the United States (US) have guidelines on hormone therapy that do not mention ovarian cancer and conclude that evidence for the increased risk of cancer due to HRT is in sufficient to make a definite recommendation. According to the guidelines in the United Kingdom (UK), such risk is only increased by prolonged use. In the case of epithelial ovarian cancer, the World Health Organization, European and US guidelines on hormone therapy suggest, that evidence for increased risk of relapse due to HRT is in sufficient to make a definite suggestion, but the rules in the UK indicate increased risk for long-term users [20].

There is insufficient data on the effect of HRT usage period on the onset and progression of ovarian cancer. The effect of some known prognostic factors, such as residual tumor and tumor differentiation during diagnosis, are more important than the duration of HRT use [21]. Despite these results, it is very likely that the heterogeneity of samples, including factors of age, stages and classifications, different treatment modalities (chemotherapy, surgery alone, radiotherapy or both) and different follow-up times, will reflect the selection bias [22].

As we know, estrogen replacement therapy (ERT) is safe in patients who have undergone surgically induced menopause by the removal of the uterus and bilateral ovaries. In order to prevent the stimulating effect of estrogen on normal and hyperplasic endometrium, several studies have added progesterone to HRT in patients with early stage EOC who protect their uterus after primary surgery [17].

With regard to duration, there is insufficient data on the effect of long or short term use of HRT on the onset or progression of ovarian cancer. A recent meta-analysis conducted by Li et al. on 1448 patients who investigated the effect of postoperative HRT on the clinical outcome of patients treated for EOC revealed that post-operative HRT did not have an impact on surveillance and recurrence (HR = 0.68, 95% CI: 0.54–0.86) [23].

Among the HRT users diagnosed with invasive EOC (n = 649) and borderline ovarian tumors (BOT; n = 150), there was no difference in 5-year survival of invasive cancer patients among HRT users and non-users. However, survival was better for those with borderline tumors who used HRT after diagnosis [24]. In addition, tumor types classified as border type, including serous and mucinous tumors had a large heterogeneity. There have been recent studies showing that borderline serous tumors can progress to low-grade serous ovarian cancer. Low-grade serous cancers are considered hormone-sensitive tumors, and therefore, it is important to avoid using HRT in patients with borderline serous tumors, although there is no definitive evidence to indicate this [25].

Evaluation of HRT after radical treatment of germ cell and cord ovarian malignancies is very important, as most of the cases are in young, premenopausal women who may be subject to several reductions in estrogen levels. However, there are no trials evaluating the use of HRT in these patients. Although HRT can be used safely for many of the germ cell tumors, we believe that it should be used carefully in a small subgroup of germ cell tumors that may secrete hormones. In the cases, the treatment of menopausal symptoms with HRT should be avoided and alternatives should be investigated after diagnosis [26].

In the foreground affects postmenopausal women, the improvement of climacteric symptoms following ovarian cancer diagnosis is an important concern for young women. Meta-analysis of 6 studies comparing 451 ovarian cancer patients who were treated with HRT after the diagnosis compared with 1070 women treated with HRT for control; revealed that there was no statistically significant difference in survival results [27, 28].

Some observational studies in this patient population have shown a possible benefit, as there is no increase in the risk of recurrence with HRT [29].

When we look at the results of two studies, which are very valuable because being prospective and evaluate according to whether or not patients with ovarian cancer receive random HRT. One of these studies was conducted on 59 patients who were received HRT with only estrogen and 66 control patients who did not receive any treatment. All stages of ovarian cancer were included in the study and the mean follow-up period was 42 months. In the group receiving HRT, the disease-free interval and OS were 34 and 44 months respectively, while in the non-treatment group, these durations were 27 and 34 months respectively, but the difference between the groups was not statistically significant [30].

For ovarian cancer, the available evidence suggests either a neutral effect on survival or a possible benefit from HRT. In view of the limitations of available evidence, factors such as the age of the patient, the presence of menopausal symptoms, and the molecular and hormonal characteristics of the tumor affect the initiation of HRT in some histological types of ovarian cancer [31].

A number of problems could not be resolved. For example, what the best HRT regimens are for patients with ovarian cancer and how long patients should take HRT after surgery, as well as how the use of HRT affects the clinical outcomes of patients with previous EOC diagnoses, require further study. At present, we know that in ovarian cancer patients there is no published study confirming the growth of microscopic residues that are encouraged by the use of HRT.

4. Cervical cancer

The mean age of cervical cancer is 48 years, and when diagnosed 70% of patients are under 54 years of age. Depending on the patient's age, the stage and histology of the tumor, such patients are usually treated with radical hysterectomies without preserving the ovarian or chemo-radiation treatment, in which patients begin to have sudden menopausal symptoms [32].

Approximately 80% of cervical cancers are composed of squamous cell carcinomas (SCC), 15% are adenocarcinoma and 5% are adenosquamous. The development of squamous cell carcinomas has never been associated with HRT. In contrast, there are studies that report the risk of adenocarcinoma of the cervix as notable in women receiving estrogen therapy (OR 2.7) [33].

In 80 patients under 45 years of age with early-stage disease treated with surgery or radiotherapy, HRT was used, while the remaining 40 cervical cancer patients were used as controls. No significant difference in survival or survival was observed between the groups [34].

5. Conclusions

According to preclinical data, estrogen and progesterone are thought to play a role in the induction and progression of endometrial cancers. When the data is examined, epithelial ovarian cancer (EOC) appears to be at least partially hormonally affected. Considering the literature, the use of HRT is controversial in gynecologic cancer survivors. Given the fear of recurrence and the risk of developing ovarian or endometrial cancer most clinicians are reluctant to write HRT prescriptions for these patients but HRT does not appear to be associated with an increased risk of relapse in ovarian and endometrial cancer survivors, especially when used for a short period of time. In order to make an inference in terms of cervical cancer, squamous cell cancer is not associated with estrogen as mentioned above, but the risk of cervical adenocarcinoma increased significantly in women receiving estrogen therapy. Prior to the decision to use HRT, it is imperative that a proper consultation is done to individualize treatment on the basis of potential risks and benefits, including close follow-ups. However, with strongly informed consent, we believe that physicians may consider writing a course of HRT treatment to minimize menopausal symptoms and illnesses related to hormonal reduction on an individual basis.

In conclusion, further studies are needed for the role of hormonal modulation in the development, treatment, and management of climacteric symptoms after diagnosis, despite the modern emphasis of precision medicine in cancer care. In the patient group diagnosed with gynecological cancer, it is necessary to better define the conditions in which HRT can provide benefit or harm. Although there are some pre-clinical and epidemiological evidence that contradicts individual experience, observational or small randomized studies, there are available data in the literature to advice women on general and specific risks and benefits of HRT. Given high discontinuation rates and low medical compliance, we still have much to do in terms of informing women about the advantages and disadvantages of HRT and encouraging the appropriate use of HRT. Finally, to the extent that we can get rid of progressive diseases such as cancer, we can achieve the expected successful healthy aging goal.

Acknowledgements

The author thanks to Assistant Prof. Dr. Nazan Ardıç who have had extensive experience and information in gynecologic field and give a great supports at the data collection stage.

Conflict of interest

The author of this manuscript declares that there is no conflict of interest.

Author details

Hasan Çilgin
Medicine Faculty, Obstetric and Gynecology Department, Kafkas University, Kars, Turkey

*Address all correspondence to: munzurluhasan@yahoo.com

References

[1] National Institutes of Health state-of-the-science conference statement: Management of menopause-related symptoms. Annals of Internal Medicine. 2005;**142**(12 Pt 1):1003-1013

[2] Noble N. Symptom management in women undergoing the menopause. Nursing Standard. 2018;**32**(22):53-63. DOI: 10.7748/ns.2018.e11041

[3] Gold EB. The timing of the age at which natural menopause occurs. Obstetrics and Gynecology Clinics of North America. 2011;**38**(3):425-440. DOI: 10.1016/j.ogc.2011.05.002

[4] Harper-Harrison G, Shanahan MM. Hormone Replacement Therapy. USA: Creighton University Omaha, StatPearls Publishing; 2018

[5] Rocca WA, Grossardt BR, Maraganore DM. The long-term effects of oophorectomy on cognitive and motor aging are age dependent. Neurodegenerative Diseases. 2008;**5**:257-260

[6] Suriano KA, McHale M, McLaren CE, et al. Estrogen replacement therapy in endometrial cancer patients: A matched control study. Obstetrics & Gynecology. 2001;**97**(4):555-560

[7] Barakat RR, Bundy BN, Spirtos NM, et al. Randomized double-blind trial of estrogen replacement therapy versus placebo in stage I or II endometrial cancer: A gynecologic oncology group study. Journal of Clinical Oncology. 2006;**24**(4):587-592

[8] Li SF, Shiozawa T, Nakayama K, Nikaido T, Fujii S. Stepwise abnormality of sex steroid hormone receptors, tumor suppressor gene products (p53 and Rb), and cyclin E in uterine endometrioid carcinoma. Cancer. 1996;**77**:321-329

[9] Aoki D. Annual report of gynecologic oncology committee, Japan society of obstetrics and gynecology. The Journal of Obstetrics and Gynaecology Research. 2014, 2013;**40**(2):338-348

[10] Biliatis I, Thomakos N, Rodolakis A, et al. Safety of hormone replacement therapy in gynaecological cancer survivors. Journal of Obstetrics and Gynaecology. 2012;**32**:321-325

[11] Yokoyama Y, Ito K, Takamatsu K, Takehara K, Nakanishi T, Harano K, et al. How do Japanese gynecologists view hormone replacement therapy for survivors of endometrial cancer? Japanese Gynecologic Oncology Group (JGOG) survey. International Journal of Clinical Oncology. 2015;**20**(5):997-1004

[12] Ayhan A, Taskiran C, Simsek S, et al. Does immediate hormone replacement therapy affect the oncologic outcome in endometrial cancer survivors? International Journal of Gynecological Cancer. 2006;**16**(2):805-808

[13] Creasman WT, Henderson D, Hinshaw W, et al. Estrogen replacement therapy in the patient treated for endometrial cancer. Obstetrics and Gynecology. 1986;**67**(3):326-330

[14] Suriano KA, McHale M, McLaren CE, et al. Estrogen replacement therapy in endometrial cancer patients: A matched control study. Obstetrics & Gynecology. 2001;**97**(4):555-560

[15] Lee RB, Burke TW, Park RC. Estrogen replacement therapy following treatment for stage I endometrial carcinoma. Gynecologic Oncology. 1990;**36**(2):189-191

[16] Guidozzi F. Estrogen therapy in gynecological cancer survivors. Climacteric. 2013;**16**:611-617

[17] Angioli R et al. Hormone replacement therapy in cancer survivors: Utopia? Critical Reviews in Oncology/Hematology. 2018;**124**:51-60

[18] Siegel RL, Miller KD, Jemal A. Cancer statistics. CA: A Cancer Journal for Clinicians. 2015;**65**:5-29

[19] Singh P, Oehler MK. Hormone replacement after gynaecological cancer. Maturitas. 2010;**65**:190-197

[20] Wentzensen N, Trabert B. Hormone therapy: Short-term relief, long-term consequences. Lancet. 2015;**385**(9980):1806-1808

[21] Zhang YL, Chen JH, Lu W, Li BL, Zhu QY, Wan XP. Efficacy of postoperative hormone replacement therapy on prognosis of patients with serous ovarian carcinoma. Chinese Medical Journal. 2016;**129**(11):1316-1321

[22] Ursic-Vrscaj M, Bebar S, Zakelj MP. Hormone replacement therapy after invasive ovarian serous cystadenocarcinoma treatment: The effect on survival. Menopause. 2001;**8**:70-75

[23] Li D, Ding CY, Qiu LH. Postoperative hormone replacement therapy for epithelial ovarian cancer patients: A systematic review and meta-analysis. Gynecologic Oncology. 2015;**139**(2):355-362

[24] Mascarenhas C, Lambe M, Bellocco R, Bergfeldt K, Riman T, Persson I, et al. Use of hormone replacement therapy before and after ovarian cancer diagnosis and ovarian cancer survival. International Journal of Cancer. 2006;**119**:2907-2915

[25] McCluggage WG. Morphological subtypes of ovarian carcinoma: A review with emphasis on new developments and pathogenesis. Pathology (Philadelphia, Pa.). 2011;**43**:420-432

[26] Biliatis I, Thomakos N, Rodolakis A, et al. Safety of hormone replacement therapy in gynaecological cancer survivors. Journal of Obstetrics and Gynaecology. 2012;**32**:321-325

[27] Singh P, Oehler MK. Hormone replacement after gynaecological cancer. Maturitas. 2010;**65**:190-197

[28] Pergialiotis V, Pitsouni E, Prodromidou A, Frountzas M, Perrea DN, Vlachos GD. Hormone therapy for ovarian cancer survivors: Systematic review and meta-analysis. Menopause. 2016;**23**:335-342

[29] Mascarenhas C, Lambe M, Bellocco R, et al. Use of hormone replacement therapy before and after ovarian cancer diagnosis and ovarian cancer survival. International Journal of Cancer. 2006;**119**:2907-2915

[30] Guidozzi F, Daponte A. Estrogen replacement therapy for ovarian carcinoma survivors: A randomized controlled trial. Cancer. 1999;**86**:1013-1018

[31] Temkin SM, Mallen A, Bellavance E, Rubinsak L, Wenham RM. The role of menopausal hormone therapy in women with or at risk of ovarian and breast cancers: Misconceptions and current directions. Cancer. 2019;**125**(4):499-514

[32] Horner MJ, Ries LAG, Krapcho M, Neyman N, Aminou R, Howlader N, editors. SEER Cancer Statistics Review, 1975-2006. Bethesda, MD: National Cancer Institute; 2009 (based on November 2008 SEER data submission, posted to the SEER website)

[33] Lacey JV Jr, Brinton LA, Barnes WA, Gravitt PE, Greenberg MD, Hadjimichael OC, et al. Use of hormone replacement therapy and adenocarcinomas and squamous cell carcinomas of the uterine cervix. Gynecologic Oncology. 2000;**77**:149-154

[34] Ploch E. Hormone replacement therapy in patients after cervical cancer treatment. Gynecologic Oncology. 1987;**26**:169-177

Chapter 7

Ovarian Hormonal Change-Related Energy Metabolism and Obesity in Menopausal Women

Jing Zhu, Mengxia Ji, Lili Xing, Zhizhi Yu, Xiaoyan Guo, Xiaopan Chen and Jing Shu

Abstract

Obesity and its related severe consequences have been a major public health problem worldwide. A significant weight gain and intra-abdominal adipose tissue accumulation are observed as women begin the menopausal transition. A number of clinical and basic research indicate that ovarian hormone may play a crucial role. However, the underlying mechanisms are largely unknown. In this chapter, we aim to systematically review the literature in the influences of ovarian hormone on the physiology of lipid and glucose metabolism, obesity-related hormone, and the regulation of body weight by the dietary intake, feeding behavior. A variety of research modalities have been used to explore the effects of MHT in perimenopausal women. Hence, we will also summarize the latest progress of MHT use on the effect of body mass, body fat redistribution, and insulin resistance, which lead to protective cardiometabolic effects.

Keywords: menopause, ovarian hormone, estrogen, metabolism, obesity, menopausal hormone therapy, adipose distribution, insulin resistance, leptin, growth hormone, dietary intake

1. Introduction

Menopause is a special period for women, which is the end of menstrual cycle and fertility and also the start of a series of changes, such as hot flashes and mood changes. Energy metabolism also changes during menopausal transition, which is important and yet does not receive enough attention. Clinical surveys observed a trend of weight gain, increased food intake, intra-abdominal fat accumulation, increased low-density lipoprotein cholesterol and triglycerides, insulin resistance, and reduced energy expedition [1, 2]. All of these changes in energy metabolism add to the risk of diabetes and cardiovascular diseases (CVDs).

The characteristic and fundamental differences in postmenopausal women are the changes in ovarian hormones. Estrogen and progesterone decreased while androgen, follicular stimulating hormone (FSH), and luteinizing hormone (LH) increased [3]. Among them, the effect of the declination of estrogen level is most studied. Estrogen receptors are expressed in various tissues, such as brain, adipose tissue, liver, and intestinal mucosa, of which all regulate energy expenditure [4]. Apart from ovarian hormones, leptin, growth hormone, and others also affect energy homeostasis and will be discussed in the text.

In this chapter, we summarize the evidence from clinical and animal studies and target to explain how hormonal changes in menopause lead to alterations in lipid

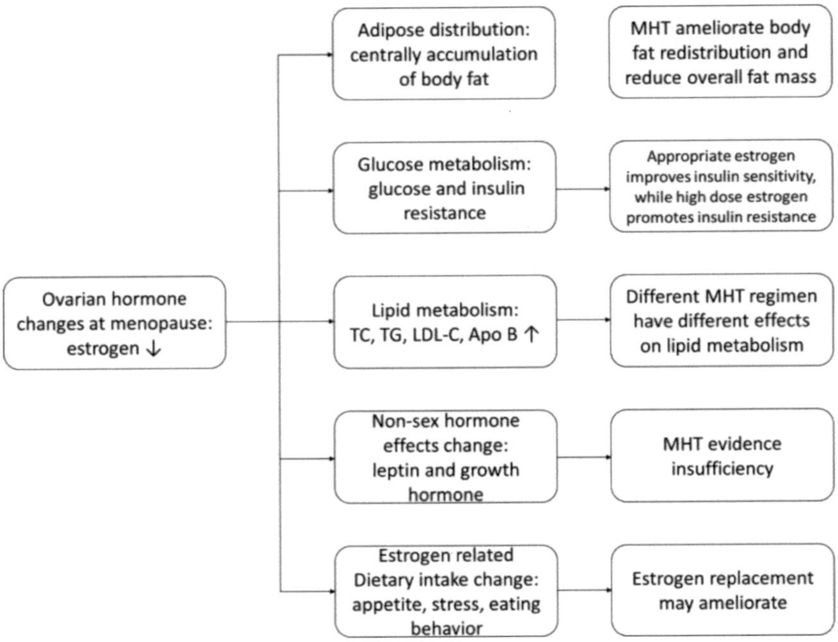

Figure 1.
Graphical overview on the contents of this chapter.

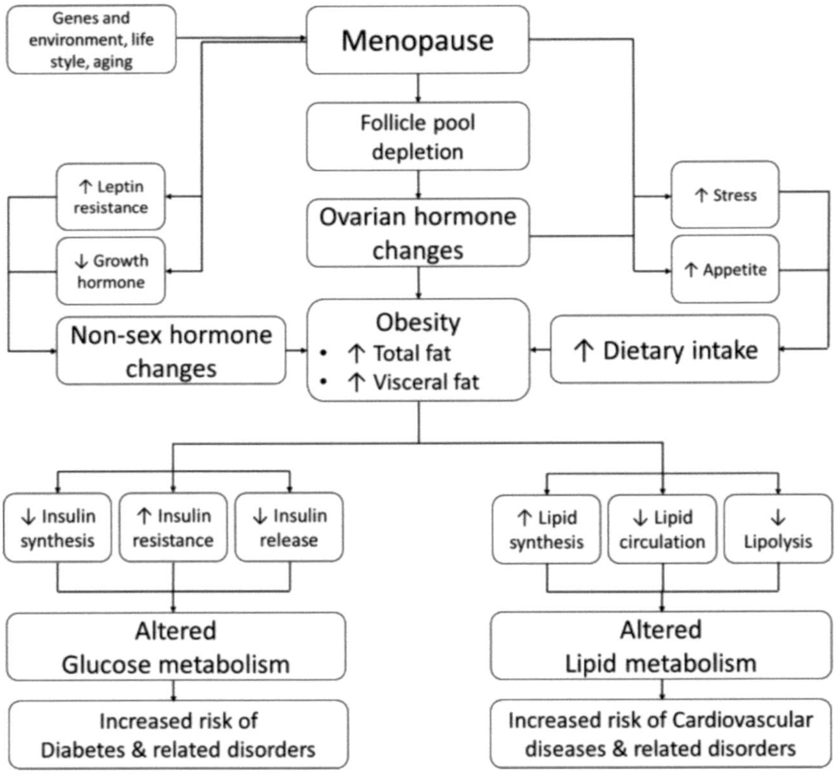

Figure 2.
Schematic illustration of possible pathophysiology underlying the ovarian hormone changes related to energy metabolism and obesity in menopause women.

and glucose metabolism, fat distribution, and food intake (**Figures 1** and **2**). We are also interested in the latest progress of the menopausal hormone therapy (MHT) and how it influences fat redistribution and metabolism (**Figure 1**).

2. Adipose distribution, metabolic consequences at menopause, and menopausal hormone therapy

2.1 The influence of menopause on adipose distribution and menopausal hormone therapy

2.1.1 Adipose distribution at menopause

The body adipose tissue distribution is different between males and females. The figure of men is pear shaped, since the adipose tissue tends to accumulate on the subcutaneous and intra-abdominal part. Whereas women's figure is apple shaped, since women's fat is more likely to accumulate on gluteal and femoral part [5]. However, mounting evidence indicated that postmenopausal women underwent deleterious changes of body adipose tissue distribution, from noncentral adiposity to central adiposity, which leads to an increased risk of CVD [6–8].

A number of factors contribute to the altered body adipose tissue distribution in postmenopausal women, including age, menopause, appetite, physical activity, and emotional changes, while age and menopause are the main reasons. A prospective study carried by Ho et al. concerning Chinese women aged 44–55 showed that the body fat percentage and central adiposity were higher among perimenopausal and postmenopausal women than that in premenopausal women [6]. Another study followed up by Caucasus and black women for 4 years and found that menopause was related to total fat increase and visceral fat increase [7]. A meta-analysis revealed that the decrease in total leg fat percentage and increase in measures of central fat were related to menopause, while increasing age was a predominant contributor [8]. This epidemiological and clinical evidence suggests that ovarian hormone may play a major role in the regulation of adipose tissue distribution.

Since 1990s, accumulating evidence suggests that androgen receptor (AR), estrogen receptor (ER), and progesterone receptor (PR) are present in adipose tissues [5]. Ovarian hormones enter the cell and bind to their specific receptors, and then the complex regulates the transcription of targeted genes. Lipoprotein lipase (LPL) is one of the most important proteins that are involved in lipid deposition. LPL is the key enzyme hydrolyzing the circulating triglycerides into glycerol and free fatty acids, which accumulate in the adipose tissues. The hormonal regulation of LPL in adipose tissues is complicated. Generally, growth hormone and estrogen inhibit lipid accumulation by suppressing the activity of LPL, while cortisol and insulin appear to exert opposite function [5].

Iverius et al. found that fasting plasma LPL activity was inversely correlated with plasma estradiol levels and positively correlated with plasma-free testosterone in obese women [9]. One study observed that when 17β-estradiol patch was placed transdermally in the gluteal region of postmenopausal women, LPL in adipose tissue from beneath was significantly decreased compared to placebo group [10]. It is also found that compared to premenopausal women, postmenopausal women have lower LPL activity in femoral adipose tissue, whereas abdominal LPL activity is comparable [11]. Palin et al. found that estrogen regulates LPL activity in a dose-dependent manner, the highest concentration of estrogen 10^{-7} mol/L significantly reduced LPL expression relative to control, while the lower concentration significantly increased LPL expression relative to control [12]. However, whether estrogen regulates LPL activity directly or indirectly remains unclear. A research from the rat model suggested that ovarian hormones exerted their regulation of LPL activity indirectly through their effect on growth hormone [13]. However, Homma and his colleagues found that estrogen markedly decreased the LPL mRNA using genetically manipulated cells and demonstrated a special sequence that was responsible for suppressing the LPL gene transcription by estrogen [14]. There might be a nongenomic mechanism existing for the regulation of ovarian hormone, which responses more rapidly, since ER was found in cellular membranes of subcutaneous abdominal and omental human adipose tissues. But the mechanism has not been completely elucidated. It appears that various components of the membrane signaling systems were involved, including the cAMP cascade and the phosphoinositide cascade [5].

2.1.2 Menopausal hormone therapy-related body fat distribution

Since the increases in total body fat and abdominal fat are associated with hormonal changes during menopause transition period, MHT may help to ameliorate the unfavorable body fat redistribution and reduce the overall fat mass.

Our team found that in ovariectomized mice, the estrogen-treated group gained less weight and had significantly lower visceral adipose mass and smaller adipocyte size than nontreated group [15]. A randomized study found that hip and abdominal circumferences and fat mass/fat-free mass ratio over the abdomen in women who received only estrogen therapy were significantly declined [16]. Postmenopausal women who used continuous combined regimen of 17-β estradiol plus norethisterone acetate showed significantly reduced central fat accumulation as assessed by waist circumference and subcutaneous abdominal fat thickness after a 6-month follow-up [17]. One study concerning the randomized controlled clinical trial of the Women's Health Initiative (WHI) showed that after 3 years of intervention with estrogen plus progestin, the treated group of women lost less lean soft tissue mass than the placebo group. Additionally, the women in the treated group had less upper-body fat distribution than the women in the placebo group [18]. Other studies compared different routes of estrogen replacement therapy and discovered that oral estrogen treatment resulted in an increase in fat mass of 5% and a decrease in lean body mass of 2%, which is equivalent to those occurring spontaneously over a 5–10-year period, whereas the transdermal estrogen did not bring a significant change in fat mass and lean mass [19, 20]. Though the conclusion is controversial, the International Menopause Society (IMS) puts it in their recommendation that menopausal abdominal fat accumulation can be ameliorated by estrogen therapy, with a reduction in overall fat mass, and maintain that a healthy diet and physical activity should also be included in weight management [21].

2.2 The influence of menopause on glucose metabolism and menopausal hormone therapy

2.2.1 Glucose metabolism at menopause

The incidence of glucose intolerance and insulin resistance increases after menopause [22]. The underlying pathogenesis of impaired glucose metabolism, although not yet fully understood, has been linked to estrogen deficiency, which is one of the characteristic changes arising with menopause. Estrogen exerts its protective effects on glycometabolism via various ways:

1. Increase insulin synthesis: Estradiol-stimulated estrogen receptor α (ERα) activates the Src/MAPK pathway, phosphorylates the transcription factor

PDX-1, and enhances NeuroD1 nuclear localization and its binding to the insulin promoter [23]. As a result, insulin gene transcription is upregulated, and insulin synthesis increased.

2. Regulate insulin release: On one hand, estrogen inhibits basal insulin secretion, which is mainly mediated by estrogen receptor β (ERβ). After an overnight fast, ERβ knockout mice carry lower blood glucose level than their counterparts in the control group and ERα gene knockout group [24]. On the other hand, estrogen promotes glucose-stimulated insulin secretion, which is mainly mediated by its plasma membrane receptor. This pathway regulates the activity of membrane-bound guanylate cyclase and activates protein kinase G. Subsequently, ATP-sensitive K^+ channels close, and calcium channels open, triggering the insulin release [25].

3. Decrease insulin-mediated glucose uptake: Study suggests that the use of estrogen or combined estrogen-progesterone therapy in women may alter glycogen synthesis, GLUT4 translocation, and other early steps in the insulin-signaling pathway, which in turn decreases whole-body glucose uptake [26].

4. Reduce insulin resistance: Low estrogen is found to be an independent predictor of insulin resistance [27]. Elevated cytosolic free calcium may be the basis of insulin resistance. It is believed that estrogen as a calcium channel blocker may reduce cytosolic calcium, antagonizing the process of insulin resistance [28].

5. Protect pancreatic β cells against inflammation-induced apoptosis: Estrogen activates Src/MAPK, PI3K/Akt signaling pathway, upregulates liver receptor homolog −1, promotes glucocorticoid synthesis, suppresses interleukin-1 and interleukin-6 transcription, and thus protects human islets against inflammation-induced apoptosis [29].

6. Reduce pro-inflammatory cytokines: Estrogen reduces pro-inflammatory cytokines in adipose tissue. It is noted that the level of TNFα, MCP-1, IL6, and macrophages increases after oophorectomy in mice [30]. By inhibiting inflammatory responses, estrogen can improve the insulin sensitivity.

After menopause, the above protective effects are impaired due to a dramatic reduction in estrogen, leading to a decreased level of insulin synthesis and glucose-stimulated secretion. At the same time, however, the inactivation and clearance of insulin are slowed in aging liver and kidney, and the serum insulin concentration exhibits an overall upward trend.

2.2.2 Menopausal hormone therapy-related glucose metabolism

MHT improves the quality of life in postmenopausal women by treating a range of symptoms with exogenous hormone supplement, using estrogen together with other hormones. However, current evidence concerning the effects of MHT on glycometabolism remains controversial.

It was found that a low estrogen status is more detrimental to glycometabolism. The second national health and nutrition survey in the United States revealed that the risk of Type 2 diabetes in postmenopausal women was significantly higher than premenopausal women. Moreover, 40~50% of menopausal women were reported to have reduced insulin sensitivity.

Further studies confirmed that estrogen has a dual effect on insulin sensitivity: appropriate estrogen improves insulin sensitivity, while high dose estrogen promotes insulin resistance. In one study, insulin tolerance test was undertaken following the estrogen replacement using conjugated equine estrogen. *K* value indicating insulin sensitivity increased by 25% with the dosage of 0.625 mg but decreased by 24.7% with the dosage of 1.25 mg [31].

Borissova et al. found that estrogen in MHT can promote insulin secretion after glucose administration, improve insulin sensitivity, and correct fasting hyperinsulinemia in postmenopausal women with Type 2 diabetes [32]. Two large randomized, double-blind trials also found that estrogen replacement significantly reduced the incidence of diabetes compared with the control group, the incidence rates were 3.5 versus 4.2% and 6.2 versus 9.5%, respectively [33, 34].

However, some scholars believe that estrogen is unfavorable for glycometabolism in view that high level of estrogen could result in a decrease in glucose tolerance in oral contraceptives users. Studies also showed that estrogen, when given beyond its physical dosage, induced the glucocorticoid secretion and thus increased the blood glucose level [35].

Lack of standardization for insulin sensitivity measurement, differences in the studied population, as well as types and routes of administration of hormone therapy may contribute to the discrepancies of effects of estrogen replacement on glycometabolism [36].

2.3 The influence of menopause on lipid metabolism and menopausal hormone therapy

2.3.1 Lipid metabolism at menopause

It is well known that estrogen has a significant effect on modulate lipid metabolism. A variety of research show that total cholesterol (TC), triglycerides (TG), low-density lipoprotein cholesterol (LDL-C), and apolipoprotein B (Apo B) increased in perimenopausal women, while menopause-related alternation in high-density lipoprotein cholesterol (HDL-C) is inconsistent [1, 37–42]. Some studies reported a significant reduction, others found an increase in menopausal transition, and rest showed no changes in HDL-C, which El Khoudary has suggested that menopause-related alterations may influence other metrics of HDL that could not be fully reflected by just the cholesterol contents of HDL particles as measured by HDL-C [43].

The underlying mechanisms that estrogen and lipid interact at a molecular level to contribute to the risk of CVD are not clear. It has been reported that estrogen-related receptor γ (ERRγ) regulates hepatic TG metabolism through the action phospholipase A2G12B [44], and polymorphic hepatic lipase is associated with estrogen modulate lipolysis of TG [45]. Della Torre et al. showed that liver ERα activity was essential for balanced lipid and TC metabolism, lack of ERα might lead to hepatic fat accumulation and nonalcoholic fatty liver disease [46]. Enza Distefano et al. suggested that estrogen activates the expression of LDL-receptor gene in HepG2 cells by tyrosine kinase signaling pathway [47]. Several research studies have suggested that estrogen can reduce circulating LDL-C but not cholesterol synthesis by downregulation of hepatic and plasma PCSK9, which is a suppressor of LDL receptors, in both animals and humans [48, 49]. Liu et al. reported that estrogen antagonizes oxidized LDL-induced secretion of macrophage matrix metalloproteinase-12 (MMP12,) and arterial stiffness that prevent from atherosclerosis in women [50].

Recent studies of our group have linked glycerol channel aquaporin 7 (AQP7) to protective effect of estrogen against body fat redistribution and hepatic steatosis in ovariectomized mice, indicating that AQP7 might be a novel checkpoint involved in the regulatory network of estrogen during menopausal obesity [15, 51]. Following up these studies, the molecular details that link AQP7 to estrogen were examined by analyzing the physical interactions between the promoter site of AQP7 and ER in our latest publication [52]. From there, we provided the first evidence that ER directly bound the estrogen response elements (EREs) in the promoter area of the Aqp7 gene and transcriptionally controlled AQP7 expression upon estrogen exposure. Therefore, there is solid ground for suggesting that Aqp7 is a direct target gene of ERs and may serve as a potential molecular target for the prevention of menopausal obesity.

In a recent study performed by Song et al., research focuses on the effects of FSH on lipid metabolism and has suggested that the marked increase of FSH expression postmenopausal combined with its receptors in liver may also reduce LDL-receptor level and subsequently result in a weakness of LDL-C endocytosis and an elevation of circulating LDL-C level [53].

Taken together, the above observations emphasize the gender differences and age independent on the lipid changes around the final menstrual period and suggest that ovarian hormone may influence the hepatic lipid synthesis, reduce the lipid circulation, upregulate the lipolysis, and lead to protective cardiometabolic effects. Growing body of literatures indicated several related functional proteins might play a crucial role in sex hormone's regulation of lipid metabolism; however, presented findings of the studies as well as the conclusion need further verification, but they are promising. Therefore, the complex association of menopause, ovarian hormone, especially estrogen, and lipid metabolism needs further extensive experimentation.

2.3.2 Menopausal hormone therapy-related lipid metabolism

Prevention of weight gain and lipid metabolic disorder is important components in the healthcare of postmenopausal women. Although the latest guideline from IMS indicated that MHT may ameliorate perimenopausal intra-abdominal fat accumulation, whether the MHT might maintain the lipid level during menopause transition has not been mentioned [21].

Numerous studies have attempted to understand the metabolic consequences of MHT use and define the effects of different MHT regimens. Major studies have consistently found MHT decrease LDL-C, TC and lipoprotein (a) levels; however, findings regarding TG and HDL-C levels have been inconsistent [45, 54–57]. Godsland reviewed the effect of different MHT regimens, estrogen alone, estrogen plus progestogen, raloxifene, or tibolone on plasma lipid and lipoprotein levels and found estrogen alone raise HDL-C and lower LDL-C and TC. Oral and transdermal estrogen had opposite effect on TG. The increases in HDL-C and TG when using estrogen alone were opposed according to the additional progesterone type. Specifically, effects arranged from the least to the greatest are dydrogesterone, medrogestone, progesterone, cyproterone acetate, medroxyprogesterone acetate, transdermal norethindrone acetate, norgestrel, and oral norethindrone acetate [58]. Stevens et al. suggested that MHT-related metabolic pathways is linked to multiple cellular processes, and the different MHT regimens might lead to distinct intracellular signal transduction events which contributed to the disparate risks for some diseases, e.g. CVD and cancer, in menopausal women with MHT [59].

In conclusion, different MHT regimens have different effects on lipid metabolism, exerting favorable and unfavorable changes. The choice for a particular regimen should consider individual demands, indications, complications, and lipid profile.

2.4 Role of nonsex hormones in energy metabolism during menopausal transition

2.4.1 Role of leptin in energy metabolism at menopause

Leptin is a protein hormone encoded by obese genes and secreted by adipose tissue. It has two effects on energy metabolism: on the one hand, it causes weight loss mainly by suppressing appetite. On the other hand, it has a number of effects on peripheral tissues: it can regulate energy balance by reducing lipid release into the blood circulation, reducing the output of triglycerides in target cells, and reducing the newly formed apolipoprotein B, which reduces the production of chylomicrons and low-density lipoprotein and increases apoA1, apoA IV, and apoE [60]. In obese people, the serum concentration of leptin is significantly elevated, which may be the result of leptin resistance [61]. At the same time, leptin plays a special role in maintaining normal reproductive function. The maintenance of human reproductive function requires adequate nutrition and storage of metabolic fuels, and leptin is a messenger with this signal [62, 63]. People who are emaciated lack such a signal.

In the peri-menopausal obesity, the role of leptin is still not clear. Several studies have found that the leptin level in the obese women was significantly higher than that in the nonobese women, but there is no significant difference in serum leptin levels pre and post menopause [64], and menopause does not significantly affect leptin production. Serum leptin levels were significantly positively correlated with BMI and waist circumference [65].

Moreover, in the studies of leptin level in different sexes, it was found that peri-menopausal women had significantly higher level of leptin than men (even after adjusting for differences in male and female body weights) [66]. In the relationship between leptin and fat mass, it is different from gender. On the one hand, it is because of the inhibitory effect of androgen in blood on leptin. On the other hand, the difference in the amount of leptin in different fat distributions may also play a role. In fact, subcutaneous fat expresses more leptin mRNA than visceral fat [67], while male subcutaneous fat is less than female, so adipose tissue in males may produce less leptin than female adipose tissue. This can explain the difference in fat content in different genders, but it cannot explain that women before and after menopause have different fat distributions but have similar leptin levels. Kastin et al. studied the transfer of peptides from the blood into the brain in mice after ovariectomy and found that the transport of leptin into the brain was lower than that before ovariectomy [68]. Thus, they suggested that the weight gain caused by the loss of ovarian function in mice might be related to the decrease in leptin transported into the brain.

2.4.2 Role of growth hormone in energy metabolism at menopause

Growth hormone (GH) levels are lower in postmenopausal women than that in premenopausal women. Postmenopausal women have changes in body weight and body fat distribution, which may also be caused by changes in growth hormone axis function [69]. Snel et al. found that the fat mass in GH-deficient adults increased, and lean mass decreased [70], and this change could be reversed after supplementation with GH, thus confirming the importance of GH in regulating fat content.

GH regulates body weight through the hypothalamic-pituitary axis. Two peptides, growth hormone releasing hormone (GHRH) and growth hormone release inhibiting hormone (GHRIH), secreted by the hypothalamus, activate and inhibit the release of pituitary GH. The stress response of GH to GHRH in postmenopausal women decreases [71]. This response is similar to that in obese and elderly population; MHT supplementation in postmenopausal women can reconstitute GH response to GHRH. This shows that the neuroendocrine release of GH plays an important role in the control of neutral steroid hormones. On the other hand, high GH concentration may have exerted negative feedback by hypothalamic GHRIH [72]. The use of arginine in postmenopausal women does reconstitute the response of GH to GHRIH [73], which has nothing to do with BMI [71]. Therefore, we can assume that obesity, menopause, and aging are the characteristics of normal neuroendocrine changes caused by excessive effects of GHRIH, but the intrinsic relationship between them remains to be further studied.

2.5 Dietary intake at menopause

Incidence of overweight and obesity is increased in perimenopausal and menopausal women, which is an important public health concern. One of the reasons for increasing obesity during the menopausal transition is the increase in food intake. A combination of biological and psychological factors exerts potent influence on the regulation of appetite and food intake.

2.5.1 Estrogen and the central control of appetite

Women during the menopausal transition had decreased estrogen. Estrogen participates in the regulation of energy homeostasis, as evidenced by an increase in food intake and obesity in ovariectomized rats. In concordance, clinical evidence showed that hunger, desire to eat, and prospective food consumption are all increased during the menopausal transition, while fasting fullness is decreased. This trend persisted in the later postmenopausal years [74]. However, both animal and human studies indicate that overeating due to the lack of estrogen can be ameliorated by estrogen replacement therapy [75].

Control of appetite is mainly performed in the hypothalamus of the central nervous system. Located in this region are arcuate, ventromedial, and paraventricular nuclei. Two major populations of arcuate neurons influence food intake in opposite directions. Neurons that extend projections to the lateral hypothalamic area express neuropeptide Y and Agouti-related peptide, which stimulate food intake and decrease energy expenditure. In other words, they extend orexigenic effects. Other arcuate neurons extend projections to the paraventricular nuclei and express proopiomelanocortin (POMC) and cocaine-amphetamine-regulated transcript (CART), which inhibit food intake and increase energy expenditure. Therefore, they extend anorexigenic effects [76, 77]. Estrogen acts as both a direct and an indirect control of appetite and food intake, modulating both anorexigenic and orexigenic signals in hypothalamus [78]. Estrogen regulates the function of the hypothalamic nuclei through complex processes. While ERα is abundantly expressed in the rodent brain in ventromedial, arcuate, and paraventricular and the medial preoptic area, ERβ expression is significantly lower [79]. Estrogens directly act on POMC neurons and regulate their cellular activity. ERα mRNA level in arcuate POMC neurons fluctuates over the course of the menstrual cycle, with the most dramatic increase on the day of proestrus, when E2 concentration is the highest [77]. In concordance, Xu et al. demonstrated that hypothalamic-specific deletion of ERa in steroidogenic factor-1 (SF1) neurons reduces energy expenditure. Deletion of ERa in POMC neurons alone increases appetite. Simultaneous deletion of ERa in POMC and SF1 neurons can add up these two effects and lead to hypometabolism and hyperphagia [80].

Peptidergic systems known to regulate ingestive behavior include ghrelin, neuropeptide Y (NPY), and melanin-concentrating hormone (MCH). Ghrelin peptide is a hunger-stimulating hormone, which is not only produced in the stomach by parietal cells but also produced in different areas of the hypothalamus, such as the aforementioned arcuate and paraventricular nuclei [81, 82]. Ghrelin regulates food intake by activating the growth hormone receptor according to the fluctuation in carbohydrate and lipid levels. Ghrelin also antagonizes the function of leptin, which promotes a sense of fullness. The antagonizing effect acts through the neuropeptide Y/Y1 receptor pathway, which increases gene expression of NPY and augment food intake [83].

NPY increases food intake potently through the function of the arcuate and paraventricular area in hypothalamus [84]. Estrogen inhibits the orexigenic activity of NPY. This inhibitory action stems from the reduced NPY mRNA expression and receptor activity by estrogen [85].

Melanin-concentrating hormone (MCH) promotes feeding behavior by direct action on the lateral nucleus in hypothalamus [86]. The arcuate and POMC neurons can stimulate the MCH activity [87]. Ovariectomized rats treated with estradiol demonstrated reduced orexigenic effect of MCH [88], which is hypothesized to be a direct effect of the reduced expression of MCH mRNA or the decreased affinity of the MCH receptor [89].

2.5.2 Stress and feeding behavior

Stress has been tied to a tendency to overeat and a preference for high-fat and high-sugar foods. Animal studies showed that chronic stress stimulates food intake and inhibits hypothalamic-pituitary-adrenal axis activity induced by acute stress [90]. In humans, food craving after stress can be predicted by high cortisol reactivity in response to stress. Epel et al. found that premenopausal women exposed to a stressful situation had higher cortisol levels and experienced higher calorie consumption, and they also tend to prefer sweets. Negative mood induced by stress also leads to greater food consumption [91]. As women experiencing menopausal transition, they are exposed to a lot of distressing symptoms, such as hot flashes, negative mood, poor sleep, recurring infections of the urogenital tract, and so on. Stress arises, which may increase their eating behavior.

Further, stress situations can decrease gastric motility. Estrogen has synergistic actions with stress mediators and interacts with neuromodulators [92]. Estrogen also influences gut function by inhibiting smooth muscle contraction. Premenopausal and postmenopausal women demonstrated a decrease in gastric motility under stress, which was similar to the general population. However, the perimenopausal women exhibited lower basal gastric motility but did not reveal a decreased gastric motility in response to stress. This indicated that many gastric changes during menopause are a rapid response to decreased estrogen levels, which happens quickly and can recover with time even without estrogen replacement [93].

Gaining better understanding of the mechanisms of increased appetite during menopausal transition promises to open novel therapeutic solutions for this population. Since the lack of estrogen plays a key role in the disturbances of food intake, MHT is one of the solutions to prevent unfavorable overeating, metabolic disturbances, and obesity.

3. Conclusions

With the aging of world population, the health issue of postmenopausal women has been unprecedented concerned. Obesity is associated with a decline of lifespan. Especially, the increased risk of weight gain, centrally accumulation of body fat, and energy metabolism disorders during the menopausal transition lead to further CVD and rise overall mortality in women. An early intervention of

MHT perimenopause is recommended, which may maintain the energy metabolic homeostasis and increase the average life expectancy. Numerous research studies have elucidated that menopause-related obesity is the combined effects of a variety of neuroendocrine and metabolic pathways, and it is well recognized that ovarian hormone plays a key role. Besides, different regimens of MHT may cause delicate difference on energy metabolism. More studies are necessary to characterize the complex effects of ovarian hormone on the energy metabolism, in which multiple organs and systems are involved.

Acknowledgements

This work was supported by grants from the National Natural Science Foundation of China [81701460 (X. C.)]; the Natural Science Foundation of Zhejiang Province [Y17H040052 (J. S)] and [LQ18H040004 (J. Z.)]; the General Research Program for Medicine and Health of Zhejiang Province [2019KY033 (J.S.)] and [2016KYA029 (J. Z.)]; and the Excellent Young Scientist Foundation of Zhejiang Provincial People's Hospital [ZRY2016A002 (X. C.)].

Conflict of interest

The authors declare no conflict of interest.

Author details

Jing Zhu, Mengxia Ji, Lili Xing, Zhizhi Yu, Xiaoyan Guo, Xiaopan Chen*
and Jing Shu*
Department of Reproductive Endocrinology, Zhejiang Provincial People's Hospital, People's Hospital of Hangzhou Medical College, Hangzhou, Zhejiang, China

*Address all correspondence to: chenxiaopan@hmc.edu.cn
and shujing@hmc.edu.cn

References

[1] Derby CA et al. Lipid changes during the menopause transition in relation to age and weight: The study of Women's health across the nation. American Journal of Epidemiology. 2009;**169**(11):1352-1361

[2] Leeners B et al. Ovarian hormones and obesity. Human Reproduction Update. 2017;**23**(3):300-321

[3] Finch CE. The menopause and aging, a comparative perspective. The Journal of Steroid Biochemistry and Molecular Biology. 2014;**142**:132-141

[4] Eyster KM. The estrogen receptors: An overview from different perspectives. Methods in Molecular Biology. 2016;**1366**:1-10

[5] Mayes JS, Watson GH. Direct effects of sex steroid hormones on adipose tissues and obesity. Obesity Reviews. 2004;**5**(4):197-216

[6] Ho SC et al. Menopausal transition and changes of body composition: A prospective study in Chinese perimenopausal women. International Journal of Obesity. 2010;**34**(8):1265-1274

[7] Lovejoy JC et al. Increased visceral fat and decreased energy expenditure during the menopausal transition. International Journal of Obesity. 2008;**32**(6):949-958

[8] Ambikairajah A et al. Fat mass changes during menopause: A metaanalysis. American Journal of Obstetrics and Gynecology. 2019. Available from: https://www.ajog.org/article/S0002-9378(19)30588-5/abstract

[9] Iverius PH, Brunzell JD. Relationship between lipoprotein lipase activity and plasma sex steroid level in obese women. The Journal of Clinical Investigation. 1988;**82**(3):1106-1112

[10] Price TM et al. Estrogen regulation of adipose tissue lipoprotein lipase--possible mechanism of body fat distribution. American Journal of Obstetrics and Gynecology. 1998;**178**(1 Pt 1):101-107

[11] Tchernof A, Despres JP. Sex steroid hormones, sex hormone-binding globulin, and obesity in men and women. Hormone and Metabolic Research. 2000;**32**(11-12):526-536

[12] Palin SL et al. 17Beta-estradiol and anti-estrogen ICI:compound 182,780 regulate expression of lipoprotein lipase and hormone-sensitive lipase in isolated subcutaneous abdominal adipocytes. Metabolism. 2003;**52**(4):383-388

[13] Vikman-Adolfsson K et al. Growth hormone but not gonadal steroids influence lipoprotein lipase and hepatic lipase activity in hypophysectomized rats. The Journal of Endocrinology. 1994;**140**(2):203-209

[14] Homma H et al. Estrogen suppresses transcription of lipoprotein lipase gene. Existence of a unique estrogen response element on the lipoprotein lipase promoter. The Journal of Biological Chemistry. 2000;**275**(15):11404-11411

[15] Jin B et al. Tissue-specific effects of estrogen on glycerol channel aquaporin 7 expression in an ovariectomized mouse model of menopause. Climacteric. 2017;**20**(4):385-390

[16] Davis SR, Walker KZ, Strauss BJ. Effects of estradiol with and without testosterone on body composition and relationships with lipids in postmenopausal women. Menopause. 2000;7(6):395-401

[17] Yuksel H et al. Effects of oral continuous 17beta-estradiol plus

norethisterone acetate replacement therapy on abdominal subcutaneous fat, serum leptin levels and body composition. Gynecological Endocrinology. 2006;**22**(7):381-387

[18] Chen Z et al. Postmenopausal hormone therapy and body composition--a substudy of the estrogen plus progestin trial of the Women's Health Initiative. The American Journal of Clinical Nutrition. 2005;**82**(3):651-656

[19] O'Sullivan AJ et al. The route of estrogen replacement therapy confers divergent effects on substrate oxidation and body composition in postmenopausal women. The Journal of Clinical Investigation. 1998;**102**(5):1035-1040

[20] dos Reis CM et al. Body composition, visceral fat distribution and fat oxidation in postmenopausal women using oral or transdermal oestrogen. Maturitas. 2003;**46**(1):59-68

[21] Baber RJ et al. 2016 IMS recommendations on women's midlife health and menopause hormone therapy. Climacteric. 2016;**19**(2):109-150

[22] Jackson RA et al. Influence of aging on hepatic and peripheral glucose metabolism in humans. Diabetes. 1988;**37**(1):119-129

[23] Wong WP et al. Extranuclear estrogen receptor-alpha stimulates NeuroD1 binding to the insulin promoter and favors insulin synthesis. Proceedings of the National Academy of Sciences of the United States of America. 2010;**107**(29):13057-13062

[24] Barros RP et al. Participation of ERalpha and ERbeta in glucose homeostasis in skeletal muscle and white adipose tissue. American Journal of Physiology. Endocrinology and Metabolism. 2009;**297**(1):E124-E133

[25] Chen ZJ, Yu L, Chang CH. Stimulation of membrane-bound guanylate cyclase activity by 17-beta estradiol. Biochemical and Biophysical Research Communications. 1998;**252**(3):639-642

[26] Rincon J et al. Mechanisms behind insulin resistance in rat skeletal muscle after oophorectomy and additional testosterone treatment. Diabetes. 1996;**45**(5):615-621

[27] Kalish GM et al. Association of endogenous sex hormones and insulin resistance among postmenopausal women: Results from the postmenopausal estrogen/progestin intervention trial. The Journal of Clinical Endocrinology and Metabolism. 2003;**88**(4):1646-1652

[28] Collins P et al. Cardiovascular protection by oestrogen--a calcium antagonist effect? Lancet. 1993;**341**(8855):1264-1265

[29] Baquie M et al. The liver receptor homolog-1 (LRH-1) is expressed in human islets and protects {beta}-cells against stress-induced apoptosis. Human Molecular Genetics. 2011;**20**(14):2823-2833

[30] Bruun JM et al. Estrogen reduces pro-inflammatory cytokines in rodent adipose tissue: Studies in vivo and in vitro. Hormone and Metabolic Research. 2003;**35**(3):142-146

[31] Lindheim SR et al. A possible bimodal effect of estrogen on insulin sensitivity in postmenopausal women and the attenuating effect of added progestin. Fertility and Sterility. 1993;**60**(4):664-667

[32] Borissova AM et al. Effect of hormone replacement therapy on insulin secretion and insulin sensitivity in postmenopausal diabetic women. Gynecological Endocrinology. 2002;**16**(1):67-74

[33] Margolis KL et al. Effect of oestrogen plus progestin on the incidence of diabetes in postmenopausal women: Results from the Women's Health Initiative hormone trial. Diabetologia. 2004;**47**(7):1175-1187

[34] Kanaya AM et al. Glycemic effects of postmenopausal hormone therapy: The heart and estrogen/progestin replacement study. A randomized, double-blind, placebo-controlled trial. Annals of Internal Medicine. 2003;**138**(1):1-9

[35] Godsland IF. The influence of female sex steroids on glucose metabolism and insulin action. Journal of Internal Medicine. Supplement. 1996;**738**:1-60

[36] Bitoska I et al. Effects of hormone replacement therapy on insulin resistance in postmenopausal diabetic women. Open Access Macedonian Journal of Medical Sciences. 2016;**4**(1):83-88

[37] Carr MC et al. Changes in LDL density across the menopausal transition. Journal of Investigative Medicine. 2000;**48**(4):245-250

[38] Matthews KA et al. Are changes in cardiovascular disease risk factors in midlife women due to chronological aging or to the menopausal transition? Journal of the American College of Cardiology. 2009;**54**(25):2366-2373

[39] Matthews KA et al. Lipid changes around the final menstrual period predict carotid subclinical disease in postmenopausal women. Stroke. 2017;**48**(1):70-76

[40] Murano T et al. Impact of menopause on lipid and bone metabolism and effect of hormone replacement therapy. The Tokai Journal of Experimental and Clinical Medicine. 2003;**28**(3):109-119

[41] Touraine P et al. New natural inactivating mutations of the follicle-stimulating hormone receptor: Correlations between receptor function and phenotype. Molecular Endocrinology. 1999;**13**(11):1844-1854

[42] Luo F et al. Estrogen lowers triglyceride via regulating hepatic APOA5 expression. Lipids in Health and Disease. 2017;**16**(1):72

[43] El Khoudary SR. HDL and the menopause. Current Opinion in Lipidology. 2017;**28**(4):328-336

[44] Chen L et al. Estrogen-related receptor gamma regulates hepatic triglyceride metabolism through phospholipase A2 G12B. The FASEB Journal. 2019;**33**(7):7942-7952

[45] Pulchinelli A Jr et al. Positive association of the hepatic lipase gene polymorphism c.514C > T with estrogen replacement therapy response. Lipids in Health and Disease. 2011;**10**:197

[46] Della Torre S et al. An essential role for liver ERalpha in coupling hepatic metabolism to the reproductive cycle. Cell Reports. 2016;**15**(2):360-371

[47] Distefano E et al. Role of tyrosine kinase signaling in estrogen-induced LDL receptor gene expression in HepG2 cells. Biochimica et Biophysica Acta. 2002;**1580**(2-3):145-149

[48] Ghosh M et al. Influence of physiological changes in endogenous estrogen on circulating PCSK9 and LDL cholesterol. Journal of Lipid Research. 2015;**56**(2):463-469

[49] Persson L et al. Endogenous estrogens lower plasma PCSK9 and LDL cholesterol but not Lp(a) or bile acid synthesis in women. Arteriosclerosis, Thrombosis, and Vascular Biology. 2012;**32**(3):810-814

[50] Liu SL et al. Cardiovascular protection in females linked to estrogen-dependent inhibition of arterial stiffening and macrophage MMP12. JCI Insight. 2019;**4**(1):122742

[51] Fu X et al. Treatment with estrogen protects against ovariectomy-induced hepatic steatosis by increasing AQP7 expression. Molecular Medicine Reports. 2016;**14**(1):425-431

[52] Xing L et al. Identification of functional estrogen response elements in glycerol channel Aquaporin-7 gene. Climacteric. 2019;**22**:1-6

[53] Song Y et al. Follicle-stimulating hormone induces postmenopausal dyslipidemia through inhibiting hepatic cholesterol metabolism. The Journal of Clinical Endocrinology and Metabolism. 2016;**101**(1):254-263

[54] Villa P et al. Low-dose estrogen and drospirenone combination: Effects on glycoinsulinemic metabolism and other cardiovascular risk factors in healthy postmenopausal women. Fertility and Sterility. 2011;**95**(1):158-163

[55] Anagnostis P et al. The effect of hormone replacement therapy and tibolone on lipoprotein (a) concentrations in postmenopausal women: A systematic review and meta-analysis. Maturitas. 2017;**99**:27-36

[56] Christodoulakos GE et al. Effect of hormone replacement therapy, tibolone and raloxifene on serum lipids, apolipoprotein A1, apolipoprotein B and lipoprotein(a) in Greek postmenopausal women. Gynecological Endocrinology. 2004;**18**(5):244-257

[57] Rossouw JE et al. Inflammatory, lipid, thrombotic, and genetic markers of coronary heart disease risk in the women's health initiative trials of hormone therapy. Archives of Internal Medicine. 2008;**168**(20):2245-2253

[58] Godsland IF. Effects of postmenopausal hormone replacement therapy on lipid, lipoprotein, and apolipoprotein (a) concentrations: Analysis of studies published from 1974-2000. Fertility and Sterility. 2001;**75**(5):898-915

[59] Stevens VL et al. Serum metabolomic profiles associated with postmenopausal hormone use. Metabolomics. 2018;**14**(7):97

[60] Stan S et al. Effect of human recombinant leptin on lipid handling by fully differentiated Caco-2 cells. FEBS Letters. 2001;**508**(1):80-84

[61] Van Doorn C et al. Leptin resistance and hippocampal behavioral deficits. Physiology & Behavior. 2017;**176**:207-213

[62] Amarase C et al. Serum leptin as a nutritional biomarker in children with cerebral palsy. The Tohoku Journal of Experimental Medicine. 2016;**239**(2):139-146

[63] Schneider JE et al. Leptin indirectly affects estrous cycles by increasing metabolic fuel oxidation. Hormones and Behavior. 1998;**33**(3):217-228

[64] Celik F, Belviranli M, Okudan N. Circulating levels of leptin, nesfatin-1 and kisspeptin in postmenopausal obese women. Archives of Physiology and Biochemistry. 2016;**122**(4):195-199

[65] Lisko I et al. Are body mass index, waist circumference and waist-to-hip ratio associated with leptin in 90-year-old people? European Journal of Clinical Nutrition. 2013;**67**(4):420-422

[66] Cundrle I Jr et al. Sex differences in leptin modulate ventilation in heart failure. Heart & Lung. 2017;**46**(3):187-191

[67] Orel M et al. Gender differences in tumor necrosis factor alpha and leptin secretion from subcutaneous and visceral fat tissue. Physiological Research. 2004;**53**(5):501-505

[68] Kastin AJ, Akerstrom V, Maness LM. Chronic loss of ovarian function decreases transport of leptin into mouse brain. Neuroscience Letters. 2001;**310**(1):69-71

[69] Fanciulli G, Delitala A, Delitala G. Growth hormone, menopause and ageing: No definite evidence for 'rejuvenation' with growth hormone. Human Reproduction Update. 2009;**15**(3):341-358

[70] Snel YE et al. Direct assessment of extracellular water volume by the bromide-dilution method in growth hormone-deficient adults. European Journal of Clinical Investigation. 1995;**25**(9):708-714

[71] Norman C et al. Estradiol regulates GH-releasing peptide's interactions with GH-releasing hormone and somatostatin in postmenopausal women. European Journal of Endocrinology. 2014;**170**(1):121-129

[72] Muller EE, Locatelli V, Cocchi D. Neuroendocrine control of growth hormone secretion. Physiological Reviews. 1999;**79**(2):511-607

[73] Gianotti L et al. Arginine counteracts the inhibitory effect of recombinant human insulin-like growth factor I on the somatotroph responsiveness to growth hormone-releasing hormone in humans. The Journal of Clinical Endocrinology and Metabolism. 2000;**85**(10):3604-3608

[74] Duval K et al. Effects of the menopausal transition on dietary intake and appetite: A MONET group study. European Journal of Clinical Nutrition. 2014;**68**(2):271-276

[75] Davis SR et al. Understanding weight gain at menopause. Climacteric. 2012;**15**(5):419-429

[76] Kozakowski J et al. Obesity in menopause - our negligence or an unfortunate inevitability? Przeglad Menopauzalny. 2017;**16**(2):61-65

[77] Hirschberg AL. Sex hormones, appetite and eating behaviour in women. Maturitas. 2012;**71**(3):248-256

[78] Butera PC. Estradiol and the control of food intake. Physiology & Behavior. 2010;**99**(2):175-180

[79] Roepke TA. Oestrogen modulates hypothalamic control of energy homeostasis through multiple mechanisms. Journal of Neuroendocrinology. 2009;**21**(2):141-150

[80] Xu Y et al. Distinct hypothalamic neurons mediate estrogenic effects on energy homeostasis and reproduction. Cell Metabolism. 2011;**14**(4):453-465

[81] Kojima M et al. Ghrelin is a growth-hormone-releasing acylated peptide from stomach. Nature. 1999;**402**(6762):656-660

[82] Nakazato M et al. A role for ghrelin in the central regulation of feeding. Nature. 2001;**409**(6817):194-198

[83] Kojima M, Kangawa K. Ghrelin: Structure and function. Physiological Reviews. 2005;**85**(2):495-522

[84] Hill JW et al. Estrogen induces neuropeptide Y (NPY) Y1 receptor gene expression and responsiveness to NPY in gonadotrope-enriched pituitary cell cultures. Endocrinology. 2004;**145**(5):2283-2290

[85] de Souza FS et al. The estrogen receptor alpha colocalizes with proopiomelanocortin in hypothalamic

neurons and binds to a conserved motif present in the neuron-specific enhancer nPE2. European Journal of Pharmacology. 2011;**660**(1):181-187

[86] Pillot B et al. Role of hypothalamic melanocortin system in adaptation of food intake to food protein increase in mice. PLoS One. 2011;**6**(4):e19107

[87] Biebermann H et al. The neuroendocrine circuitry controlled by POMC, MSH, and AGRP. Handbook of Experimental Pharmacology. 2012;**209**:47-75

[88] Messina G et al. Hormonal changes in menopause and orexin-a action. Obstetrics and Gynecology International. 2013;**2013**:209812

[89] Nahon JL. The melanocortins and melanin-concentrating hormone in the central regulation of feeding behavior and energy homeostasis. Comptes Rendus Biologies. 2006;**329**(8):623-638

[90] Tryon MS, DeCant R, Laugero KD. Having your cake and eating it too: A habit of comfort food may link chronic social stress exposure and acute stress-induced cortisol hyporesponsiveness. Physiology & Behavior. 2013;**114-115**:32-37

[91] Epel E et al. Stress may add bite to appetite in women: A laboratory study of stress-induced cortisol and eating behavior. Psychoneuroendocrinology. 2001;**26**(1):37-49

[92] Meleine M, Matricon J. Gender-related differences in irritable bowel syndrome: Potential mechanisms of sex hormones. World Journal of Gastroenterology. 2014;**20**(22):6725-6743

[93] Huerta-Franco MR et al. Gastric responses to acute psychological stress in climacteric women: A pilot study. Menopause. 2019;**26**(5):469-475